OSCEOLOGIST
HIGH YIELD IMAGES and TOPICS for OSCE

EDITOR
Hamad Almutairi
Final Year Medical Student Royal College of Surgeons in Ireland


All rights reserved. Any part of this book may not be reproduced or used in any manner without permission of the editor.


The editor is not responsible for any injuries caused due to using this book. All suggestions and comments are welcome contact by email : osceologist@outlook.com

PREFACE
Learn from everything. Respect everyone. Improve yourself

I hope you find this book helpful

This book is dedicated to Ireland & Kuwait

# Contents

Breast Examination ................................................................. 3

Thyroid Examination .............................................................. 14

Cardio Examination ................................................................ 29

Respiratory Examination ........................................................ 46

GIT Examination .................................................................... 57

Hernia & Stoma Examination ................................................. 69

Venous Vascular Examination ................................................ 78

Arterial Vascular Examination ............................................... 83

Shoulder Examination ............................................................ 90

Hand Examination .................................................................. 98

Hip Examination ..................................................................... 115

Knee Examination .................................................................. 124

Spine Examination ................................................................. 132

Upper Limb Neurological Examination ................................. 134

Lower Limb Neurological Examination ................................. 144

Cranial Nerve Examination .................................................... 152

Parkinson Examination .......................................................... 168

Acromegaly Examination ....................................................... 176

Cushing Examination ............................................................. 179

Renal Examination ................................................................. 181

# Breast Examination

| | |
|---|---|
| **General** | 1. Wash hands, introduce yourself, get name and age, explain your roles and gain permission<br>2. Chaperone or female nurse<br>3. Top off, setting on side of bed<br>4. Where is the complaint from Left or right breast? |
| **Inspection** | 1. Around the bed<br>2. patient (metastasis SXS: dyspnea, dysphonia, ascites, weight loss, cachexia and jaundice)<br>3. Breast and axilla:<br>A. Symmetry, Lump, dimpling (cooper ligament), and retraction<br>B. Skin changes:<br>• ulceration(cancer)<br>• scar (mastectomy)<br>• erythema: peau d'orange, prominent blood vessel (malignant), acute mastitis (breast fed, S.aureus) and breast abscess.<br>C. Skin thickening with prominent pores(cancer)<br>D. Nipple:<br>• Asymmetry, inverted and retracted (malignant)<br>• Scaling, Rash and ulcer (Paget disease or eczema)<br>• **Discharge:**<br>- Blood from single duct: cancer, intraductal papilloma(benign)<br>- Milk: galactorrhea<br>- Serous: fibrocystic<br>- Greenish: ductal ectasias<br>- Purulent: abscess<br>4. Ask patient to press hip, raise hands above head, lean forward while hands above head to elicit dimpling, asymmetry |
| **Palpation:**<br>1. Lying supine with the examined side hand behind head<br>2. Start with healthy side while | 1. Palpate clockwise with the three middle fingers starting from upper outer quadrant in circular motion including nipple and axillary tail:<br>• **light and deep palpation If you notice lump:**<br>4S,4Tb, FCM<br>- Site<br>- Size<br>- Shape<br>- Surface (nodular, smooth, irregular)<br>- Border (well, poor defined)<br>- Temperature (back of hands)<br>- Transillumination<br>- Tenderness (watch pt. face) |

# Breast Examination

| | |
|---|---|
| the other covered | - Mobility<br>- Consistency (soft, rubbery, firm, hard)<br><br>▪ **Fixity (infiltration of tumor):**<br>a) **Skin** (unable to pinch up the skin away from tumor).<br>b) **Pectoral muscle** (try to move the lump with your fingers then ask press hip if the lump mobility is restricted then it's fixed to muscle)<br>c) **Breast tissue** (stabilize the breast with one and move the tumor with other (fibroadenoma freely movable, caner not<br>d) **Chest wall:** immobile at all<br><br>2. Squeeze the nipple (send discharge to cytology)<br>3. Palpate (rolling movement): axillary lymph, Cervical and supraclavicular lymph nodes (patient arm should be rested in your arm and warn the patient might be uncomfortable)<br>*firm non tender slowly progressive (cancer)<br><br>➢ **Axillary lymph groups:**<br>1. Pectoral(anterior) (main drainage from breast) palpate posterior surface of pectoralis major muscle while the other hand supporting the anterior surface of pectoralis major<br>2. Subscapular (posterior): behind Patient palpate the posterior axillary fold muscle.<br>3. Humeral(lateral) with both hands palpate the upper humeral head<br>4. Central (basal) compress armpit skin above the chest wall<br>5. Apical behind clavicle: palpate deep in armpit while the other is supraclavicular fossa |
| The End | 1. **Examine for metastasis:** lung (pleural effusion, consolidation), GIT(hepatomegaly), spine(tenderness)<br>2. **Rule out metastasis:**<br>▪ Blood: LFT, hypercalcemia (bony met)<br>▪ Imaging (chest, abdominal) bone scan<br>▪ Ultrasound for ovary (krukenberg tumor: transcoelomic spread to ovary)<br>▪ Ask patient to cover up and do complete triple assessment (lump) |

❖ **Lymph drainage:**
a. **Laterally(major):** Axillary lymph nodes Which has three levels in relation to pectoralis minor:
- **One**: below

# Breast Examination

- **Two**: underneath
- **three**: above
b. **Medially:** internal mammary nodes

### ❖ Triple assessment:
I. **Physical examination**
II. **Imaging:**
   1. **Mammography:**
      - Older women, 2 views (MLO, CC)
      - Cancer: micro Calcifications, irregular asymmetrical density, speculation (upper outer quadrant)
      - **\*risk assessment by scoring system BI-RADS**
   2. **MRI:**
      - High risk patients and younger women (dense breast)
   3. **US:** for under **35** years
      - **Cancer**: solid irregular outline
      - **Cyst**: smooth outline
III. **Fine needle aspiration cytology** (FNAC), or core needle biopsy (tissue) or open biopsy, FNA (c1 to c5)
   C1 - Inadequate
   C2 - Benign
   C3 - Equivocal (Atypical cells)
   C4 - Suspicious
   C5 – Malignant
   *core biopsy tells if in situ carcinoma or infiltrating carcinoma and receptor status

- **Risk Factors:**
(Tool to assess Risk factor: Gail model, Claus model, BRCApro)

- **Description**

| Fibrocystic Breast (30-50) | Fibroadenoma (Younger) | Cancer (Elderly) | Differential Diagnosis |
|---|---|---|---|
| - Bilateral well defined<br>- Round smooth Rubbery<br>- Transient cyclic pain and tenderness | - Single or multiple well defined round<br>- Smooth firm or, rubbery and mobile (breast mouse)<br>- *less than 5 cm (size changes over menstrual cycle) | - Irregular<br>- Firm<br>- Painless<br>- Fixed | - Lipoma<br>- Hamartoma<br>- Sebaceous cyst<br>- Fat necrosis (trauma)<br>- Phyllodes tumor<br>- Solitary cyst (well defined smooth firm). |

## Breast Examination

### ❖ Types of breast cancer:
**A. Noninvasive:**
1. **Ductal:** comedo necrosis (high grade), visible in mammogram
2. **Lobular:** bilateral, multifocal, impalpable and invisible mammogram

**B. Invasive:**
1. Ductal (common)
2. Lobular
3. Mucinous
4. Medullary
5. Inflammatory: painful, Invasion of dermal lymphatics (peau d' orange)

- **Prognosis (survival):**

Nottingham prognostic index(NPI) = [0.2 x Size(cm)] + Nodes + Grade
1. Staging (TNM especially lymph node positive)
2. Grading (Bloom-Richardson system)
3. Her2 over-expression worst
4. ER or PR negative worst
5. Ki67 division score and S fraction score
6. Triple negative high met, recur poor prognosis

### ❖ Treatment:
- **Surgeries:**
1. **Breast-conserving therapy** (lumpectomy) for monocentric, less than 4 cm:
   - wide local excision usually followed with radiation to reduce recurrence (whole breast irradiation or APBI) on prone position (decrease ration to nearby organs)

\* Subareolar tumors(difficult), previous radiation to thorax, pregnancy and diffuse calcification are contradictions

2. **Mastectomy:** multicentric, small breast, more 4 cm tumors and DCIS
   a. Simple (breast tissue)
   b. Total mastectomy
   c. Skin-sparing and nipple sparing
   d. Mastectomy with immediate reconstruction
   e. Radical mastectomy (breast tissue +pectoralis major, minor axillary lymph nodes) if modified (Patey)all removed except pectoralis major.

- **Complications:**
- Winged scapula (internal thoracic nerve)
- Intercostobrachial neuralgia
- Post mastectomy pain syndrome
- Axillary vein thrombosis
- Seroma, lymphedema, infection, bleeding

# Breast Examination

- **Breast reconstruction: immediate or delayed**
  - **For example:** Becker implant (under pectoralis muscle), DIEP, TRAM, LD flap

- **Chemotherapy:**

Preoperative to reduce size for met ,lymph positive , large size
- **For example:** CMF, CAF, MMM regime
- **Side effects:** Allopica, marrow depression and N/V

- **Hormone therapy:**
1. HER2-targeted therapy (Trastuzumab) SE :CHF so Do Echo before administration
2. Tamoxifen(antiestrogen) for premenopausal (ER + and PR +) might add Oophorectomy
- **Side effects:** endometrial cancer, blood clotting (PE and stroke), tamoxifen flare)
3. Aromatase inhibitor (anastrozole) for postmenopausal (ER+)
4. premenopausal and an ER+ve tumor : ovarian ablation (via surgery or radiotherapy)

**Radiotherapy :**
After wide local excision , Lymph positive ,large size

- **Lymph Node Removal**
- Sentinel lymph node if positive **(>2mm)** do axillary lymph node clearance
- **Side effects:** lymphedema (progress to Stewart-Treves syndrome) and Intercostobrachial neuralgia
- Lymphedema reduced by:
- Weight loss
- Elevate arm
- Manual compression
- Elastic sleeve
- Diuretic
- Avoid blood pressure cuff and needle

- **Metastasis Management:**
- Bone (Bisphosphonates, radiation)
- Pleural effusion (pleural drainage)
- Radiotherapy for bony metastasis

# Breast Examination

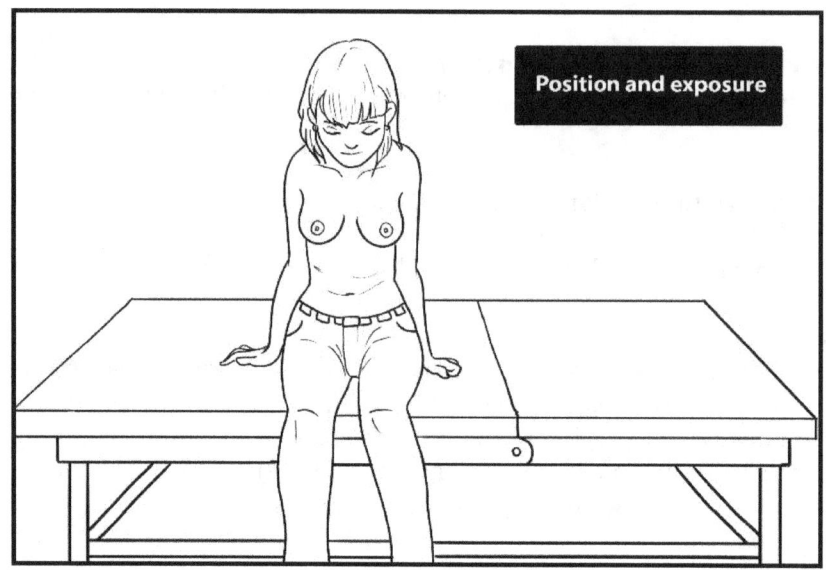

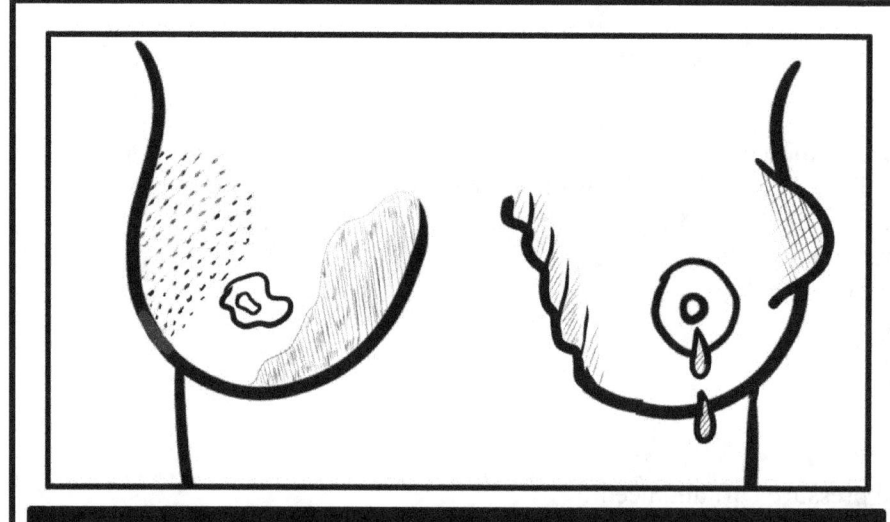

**Left breast:** nipple discharge, lump and dimpling
**Right breast:** peau d'orange, erythema, and Paget disease

# Breast Examination

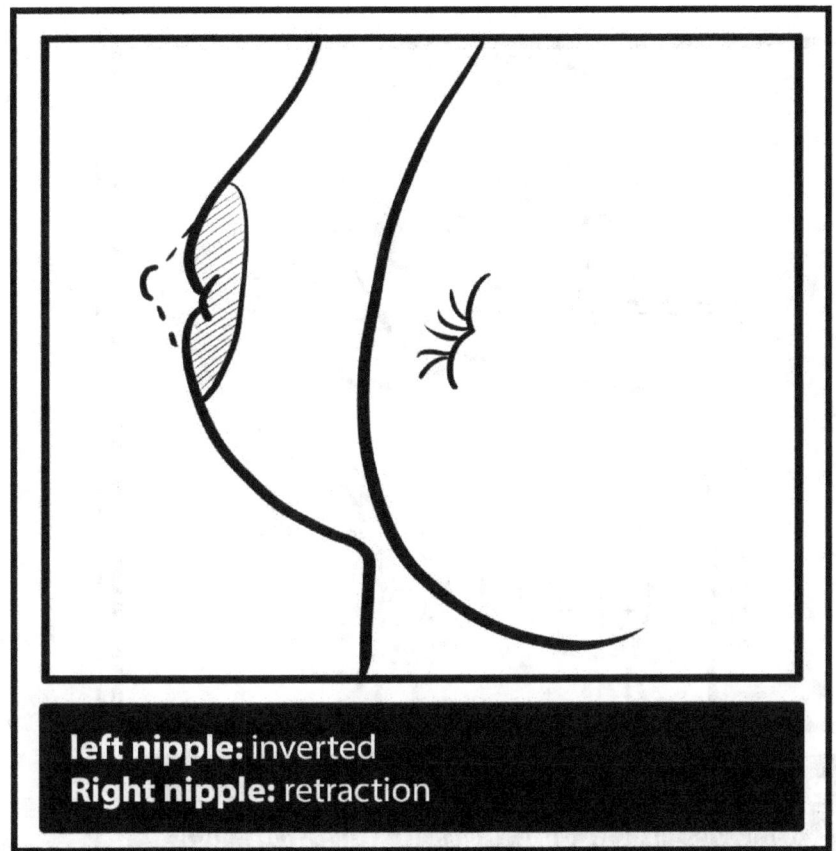

**left nipple:** inverted
**Right nipple:** retraction

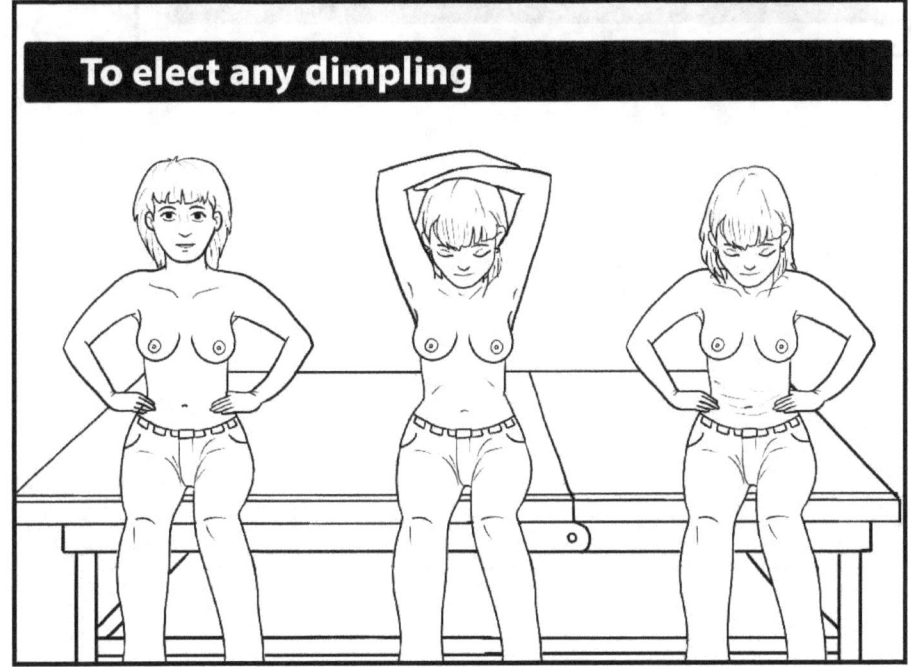

To elect any dimpling

**Breast Examination**

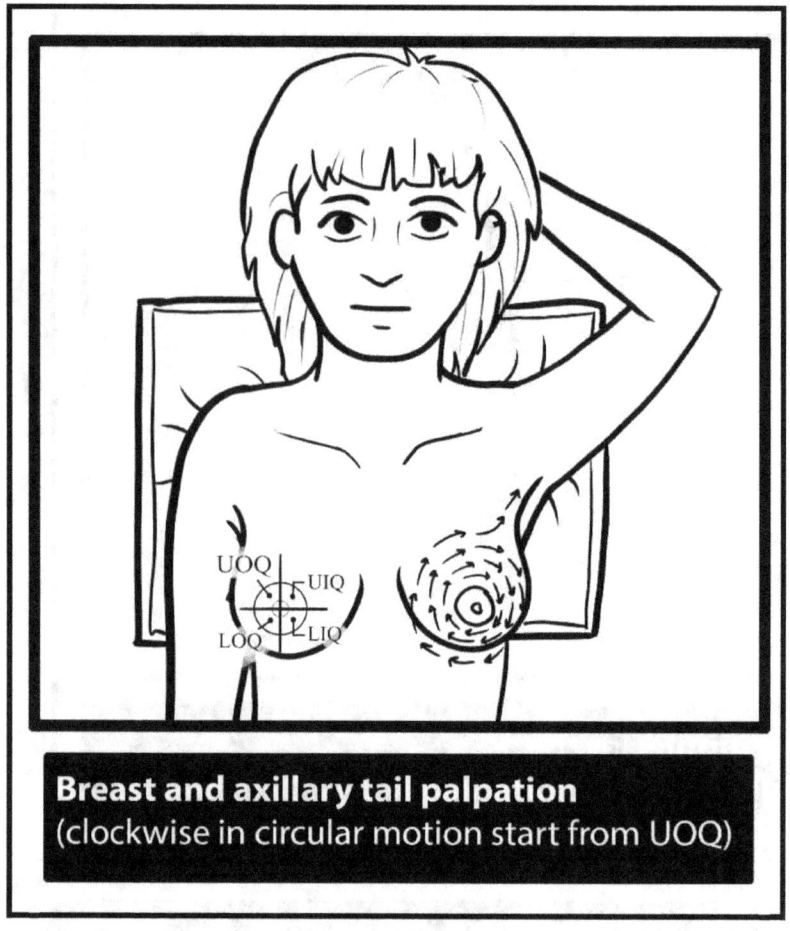

**Breast and axillary tail palpation**
(clockwise in circular motion start from UOQ)

**Breast Examination**

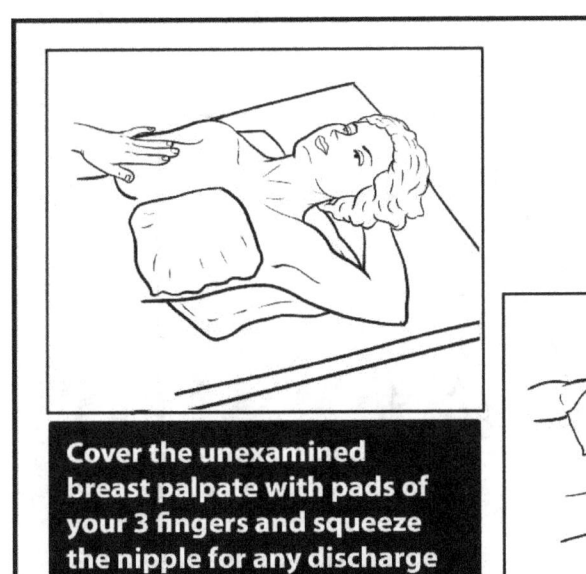

Cover the unexamined breast palpate with pads of your 3 fingers and squeeze the nipple for any discharge (or just ask)

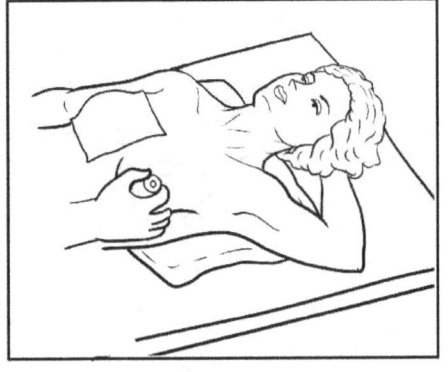

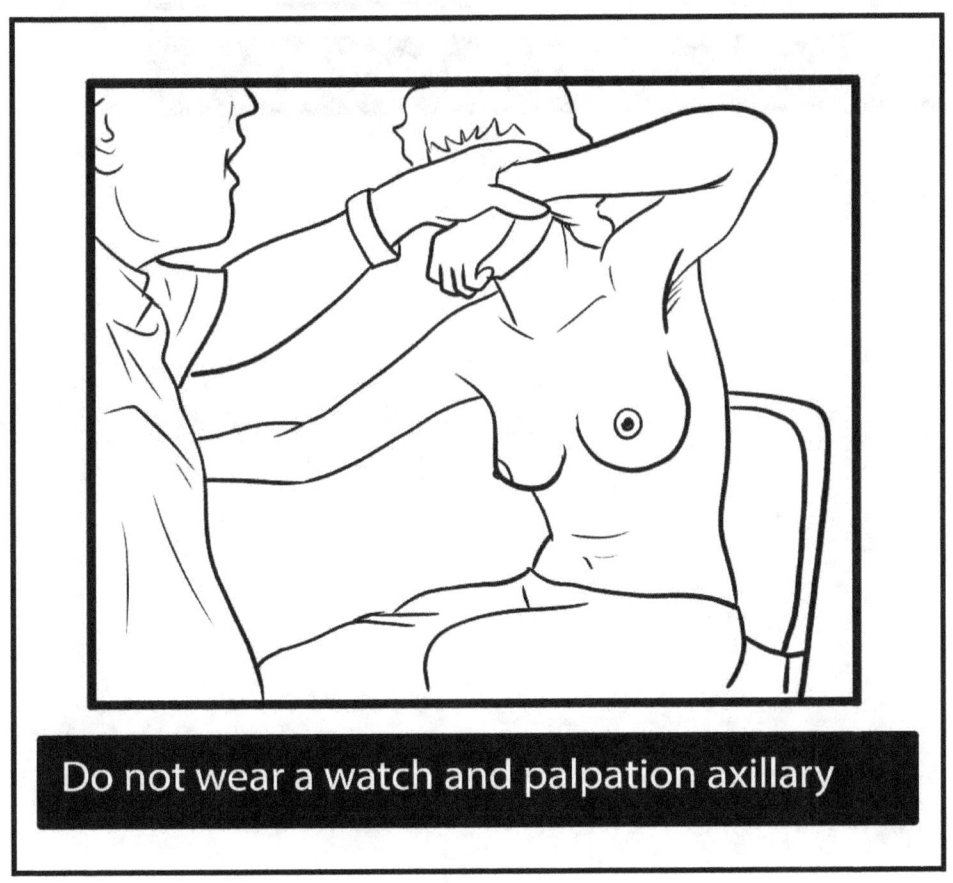

Do not wear a watch and palpation axillary

# Breast Examination

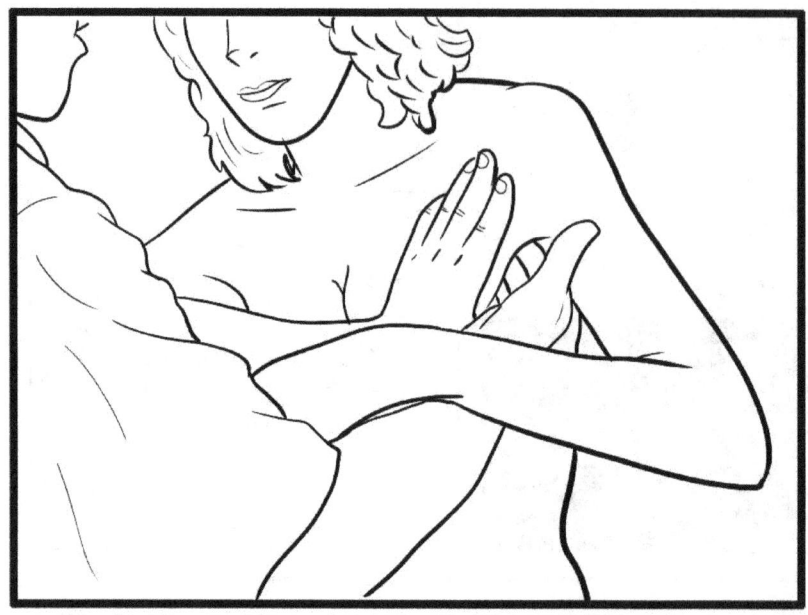

**Pectoral** (anterior)

# Breast Examination

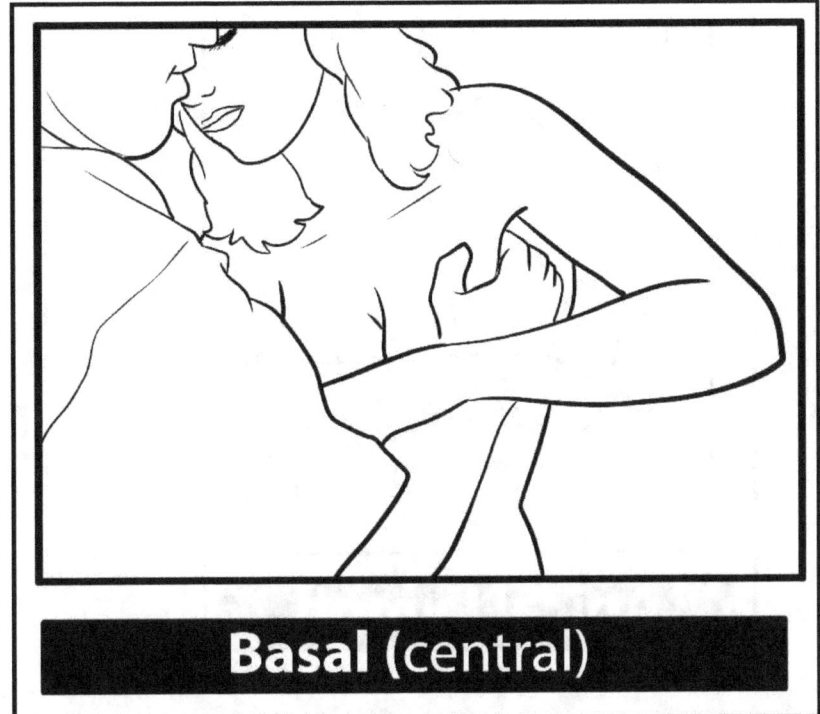

**Basal** (central)

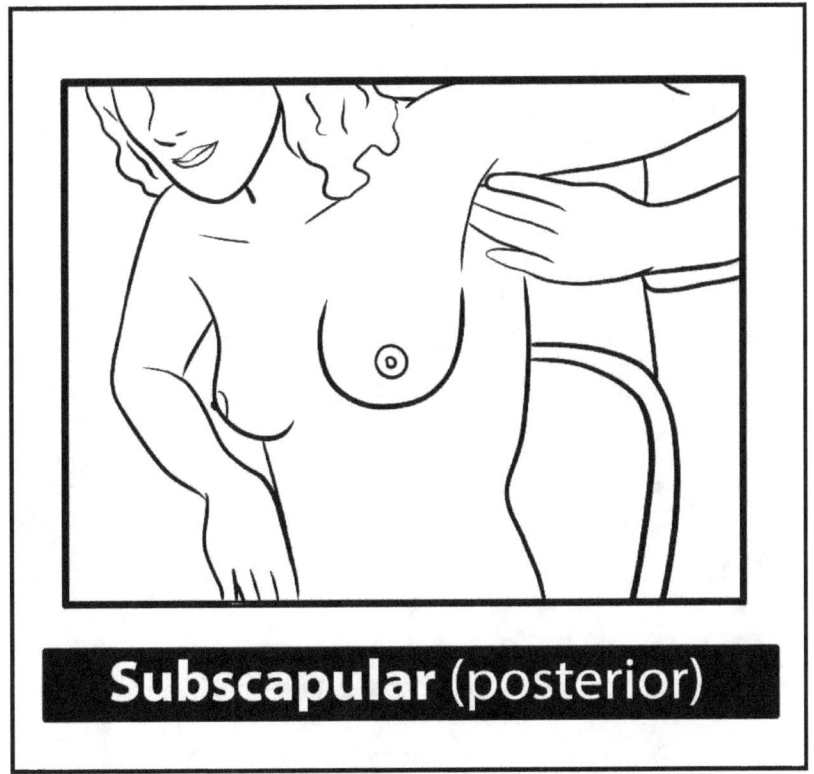

**Subscapular** (posterior)

**Breast Examination**

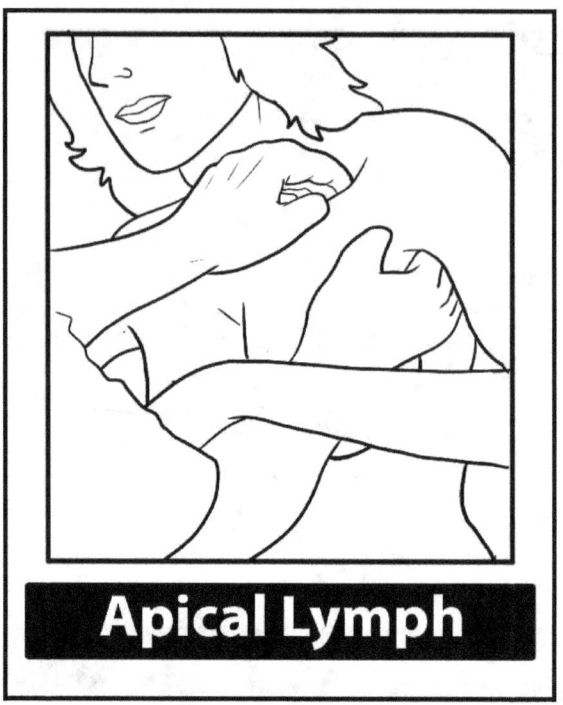

# Thyroid Examination

| | |
|---|---|
| **General** | 1. Wash hands, introduce yourself, get name and age, explain your roles and gain permission<br>2. Patient seated in a chair with exposed neck |
| **Inspection** | 1. **Around the patient (medicine)**<br>2. **Patient**:<br>- BMI<br>- Clothing appropriate to weather<br>- agitated, restless(hyperthyroidism)<br>- Lethargic, hypoactive(hypothyroidism)<br>- Hoarseness, dyspnea, stridor (Retrosternal goitre, malignant signs)<br><br>3. **Hands:(TTV SO PPP)**<br>• Thyroid acropachy/clubbing (Graves' disease)<br>• Temperature: (cold and dry hypothyroidism, hot hyperthyroidism)<br>• Vitiligo (autoimmune thyroiditis+++Hashimoto )<br>• Hyperthyroidism:<br>- Moist and warm hands (feel the palm)<br>- Onycholysis (Plummer's Nails):separation of nails bed<br>- Palmar erythema<br>- Postural fine tremor: paper above outstretched hands<br>• Radial Pulse:(tachycardia, AFib in hyperthyroidism), (bradycardia in hypothyroidism)<br>• Carpal tunnel syndrome: thenar atrophy , Tinel and Phalen tests(hypothyroidism)<br><br>4. **Face**:<br>• Horner's syndrome (malignant tumor, large goitre)<br>• Thin coarse hair + bilateral loss of outer ⅓ eyebrow + round face +puffy eye + facial myxedema (hypothyroidism)<br>• Graves ophthalmopathy:<br>a. Exophthalmos or Proptosis: (look from above) may be unable to close eyes<br>▪ **DD**:<br>- Orbital tumor, cavernous sinus thrombosis<br>b. Chemosis, conjunctivitis, ulceration<br>c. Ophthalmoplegia: H test<br>- diplopia, pain, restriction of eyes movements (Inferior rectus followed by medial, superior, levator and lateral rectus.)<br>d. Stellwag's sign: few blinkings |

## Thyroid Examination

| | |
|---|---|
| | **Other signs that associated with thyrotoxicosis:**<br>- Upper eyelid retraction (sclera above cornea visible)<br>- **Lid lag test:**<br>- Patient head still<br>- ask pt to follow your index with his eyes<br>- Move your index up and down<br>- Notice any sclera visible above corna<br><br>**5. Neck (front, sides):**<br>- Thyroidectomy Scars(very thin ,might have erythema , if you suspect it and on palpation you do not feel thyroid lobe then it's a scar )<br>   Indications (cosmetic cancer, refractory hyperthyroidism fail to respond to medication, retrosternal goitre<br>- Prominent vein(thoracic inlet obstruction<br>- Obvious midline swelling: symmetrical, asymmetrical nodules (single, multiple),<br>- Sip of water (move with swallowing: thyroid pathology)<br>- Stick tongue out: thyroglossal cyst elevates, |
| **Palpation** | 1. Palpate with fingers pads while standing behind the patient and slightly flex the neck<br>- Lump (describe as in breast lump) (describe each lobe affected)<br>- Palpable the lower border to rule out retrosternal goitre)<br>- Sip of water: While hand on lump<br>* **Grave:** nontender diffuse smooth symmetrical enlargement<br>* **Multinodular toxic goitre:** multinodular asymmetrical enlargement<br>* **Tenderness:**<br>- Viral thyroiditis, De Quervain's (subacute) thyroiditis<br>* Cancer:—fixed(tethered ), palpable lymph nodes, vocal cord paralysis, hard,<br>- Diffuse Enlargement (grave, Hashimoto, endemic, euthyroid like acromegaly ,idiopathic )<br>- Nodular (cancer, toxic multinodular goitre, adenoma)<br>2. Head and neck lymph nodes<br>- Delphian node (prelaryngeal lymph node) the first lymph that thyroid cancer metastasis<br>3. Tracheal deviation (retrosternal goitre) |

## Thyroid Examination

| | | |
|---|---|---|
| **Percussion** | - | Manubrium sterni dullness indicates retrosternal goitre |
| **Ausculte** | - | Over both thyroid lobes for Bruit (grave disease) |
| **Other** | | <ul><li>Proximal myopathy (hypothyroidism, hyperthyroidism), standing from chair with crossed arm</li><li>Knee reflex:</li></ul>- slow relaxing reflex (hypothyroidism)<br>- brisk(hyperthyroidism)<ul><li>Pretibial myxoedema (Graves' disease)</li><li>Non-pitting oedema (hypothyroidism)</li><li>Pemberton's sign (retrosternal goitre):</li></ul>- Ask the patient to raise both arms up<br>- Notice any the face for plethora(redness), cyanosis and look at the neck for vein distention<br>- Ask the Pt to take a deep breath in (inspiratory stridor) (thoracic inlet obstruction from retrosternal goitre)<ul><li>Kocher's test (tracheal compression by malignant tumor, multinodular goitre, retrosternal goiter)</li><li>Berry sign (absence of carotid pulse due malignant tumor)</li><li>Non-pitting in lower limb oedema Hypothyroidism</li><li>If you notice thyroidectomy scar offer to :To check hypoparathyroidism signs: Chvostek's or Trousseau's</li><li>Examine scalp any bony lump (follicular carcinoma met by blood to bone)</li><li>Cardiac auscultation for :systolic flow murmurs or CHF(bibasal; crepitation )seen in high output failure due to hyperthyroidism</li></ul> |
| **The End** | | - Do cardiac (high-output heart failure)<br>- Solitary thyroid nodule (FNA biopsy, thyroid scan, ultrasound)<br>- Thyroid function test<br>- Laryngoscopy:(RLN palsy)<br>- CT, X-ray (tracheal compression) |

## Thyroid Examination

| Solitary thyroid nodules(STN) | Multinodular Goiter (secondary thyrotoxicity) | Diffuse goitre (primary thyrotoxicity) |
|---|---|---|
| 1. Elderly Female<br>2. Due:<br>**A. Benign**<br>• Follicular adenoma (no capsular and vascular invasion)<br>• Thyroiditis<br>• Cyst<br>• Dominant Nodules in multinodular goitre<br>**B. malignant** (Carcinoma) | Middle aged female<br>**Due:**<br>• Iodine deficiency<br>• Goitrogens Heredity<br>• **Features:**<br>a) Afib + heart failure (common)<br>b) Eyes symptoms not common<br>c) Mild Hyperthyroidism<br>d) nodules overactive<br>e) Patchy uptake (radioiodine uptake)<br>f) Surgery only (total+subtotal thyroidectomy)<br>**complications:**<br>a) Toxicity (Plummer syndrome)<br>b) Malignancy<br>c) Retrosternal extension | 1. Young female<br>2. **Due:**<br>• **Graves' disease**<br>• **Features**:<br>a) No cardiac features<br>b) Eyes symptoms (common)<br>c) thyroid-stimulating immunoglobulins and antibody<br>d) Severe Hyperthyroidism<br>e) diffuse uptake (radioiodine scan)<br>f) All types of treatment |

- **Grades (WHO) of Goitre:**

(1) = Not palpable/nor visible
(2) = Only palpable/not visible
(3) = Visible

- **Investigations for nodules:**
1. **FNAC classification: cells**
1. Non-diagnostic or unsatisfactory
2. Benign
3. Atypia of undetermined significance (AUS) or follicular lesion of undetermined significance (FLUS)
4. Follicular neoplasm or suspicious for a follicular neoplasm;

# Thyroid Examination

5. Suspicious for malignancy
6. Malignant

* **Core-needle or open biopsy: for follicular carcinoma(not FNA because it will not be able to distinguish between follicular ca where here vascular and capsular invasion and adenoma)**
1. **Thyroid scan:** cold nodule (malignant), hot(benign)
2. **US:**
- **Malignant:** solid, hypoechoic, irregular border
- **Benign:** cyst, hyperechoic, well-defined border

- **Carcinoma:**
- features in favour of malignant nodules:
- Male
- Extremes of age younger than 20 years, older than 70
- Nodule:
a. Single rapidly growth fixed(does not move with water sipping)
b. Firm consistency
c. Irregular
d. Previous radiation the neck
e. Local invasion :Vocal cord paralysis (recurrent laryngeal nerve paralysis),dysphagia
f. Cervical LDP
g. Elevated serum calcitonin
h. Family history of thyroid cancer

- **Prognosis:**
- **Prognostic schemes: GAMES** scoring (PAPILLARY & FOLLICULAR CANCER)
- **G** Grade
- **A** Age of patient when tumor discovered
- **M** Metastases of the tumor (other than Neck LN)
- **E** Extent of primary tumor
- **S** Size of tumor (< 5cm)
- The patient is then placed into a high or low risk category

- **Risk Factors:**
- Radiation (**Papillary** ca)
- Autoimmune thyroiditis
- Genetic (**MEN** type 2, Cowden Syndrome)

- **Tumor marker:**
1. Thyroglobulin(papillary & follicular)
2. calcitonin( medullary)
3. RET proto-oncogene mutation (medullary)

## Thyroid Examination

4. If suspect Medullary :men2b syndrome remember to check for pheochromocytoma before you do the surgery and treat it(Plasma metanephrine testing &24-hour urine collection assessment of catecholamines ,metanephric

- **Treatment :**
- **Total Thyroidectomy :**
  - cancers ≥4 cm & extrathyroidal extension, or metastases to lymph nodes or distant sites
  - Unilateral lobectomy smaller intrathyroidal tumors
    Regional neck dissection : LPD(+)
  - Central(level 1),Lateral(level 2,3,4)

- **Radioactive iodine (I131) ablation**
- **Post-surgery : levothyroxine therapy**

- **Types of thyroidectomy**
  - Thyroid lobectomy (single lobe +/-isthmus)
  - Near total thyroidectomy(whole thyroid except <1 g left, No risk for RLN )
  - total thyroidectomy(whole thyroid ,risk for RLN)
  - Subtotal thyroidectomy(whole thyroid except <8 g, to achieve euthyroid state and avoid lifelong thyroid hormone replacement)
  - Hartley–Dunhill procedure

- **Complications:**

- Hypoparathyroidism
  - Hypocalcemia :tetany, prolonged QT interval
  - Chvostek's sign (facial muscle spasm by tapping on the facial nerve
  - Trousseau sign (carpopedal spasm when a blood pressure cuff are inflated ,paresthesias: numbness of perioral or hands
  - Give IV calcium and IV vit D

- Hypothyroidism (Oral thyroxine)
- Thyroid storm
- Recurrent laryngeal nerve palsy unilateral(hoarseness),bilateral RLN Injury necessitates tracheostomy)
- +sympathetic nerve chain (Horner syndrome),superior laryngeal palsy(low tone, weak)
- Infection ,hematoma(stridor),tracheal damage

## Thyroid Examination

| Papillary (80%) | Follicular 15% | Medullary 5% | Anaplastic 1% |
|---|---|---|---|
| - **Histology**: Orphan Annie + psammoma body<br>- Met to Cervical Lymph<br>- Good prognosis unless Tall cell variety, Columnar cell.<br>- Hemithyroidectomy and isthmectomy (small size)<br>- Total thyroidectomy for (bilateral, previous radiation, metastasis)<br>- Lymph dissection (lymph positive)<br>- Radioiodine therapy<br>- High thyroglobulin after surgery indicate recurrence<br><br>* 'Lindsay tumor | - Met by blood<br>* Hürthle cell cancer mets by blood and lymph<br>- Bad prognosis (vascular and capsular invasion)<br>- Total thyroidectomy<br>- Radioiodine therapy | - Met by lymph<br>- Histology: Amyloid stroma<br>- C-cells (parafollicular cells)<br>- Secrets calcitonin (Diarrhea, face flushing)<br>- MEN syndromes: IIa and IIb<br>- Total thyroidectomy<br>- Lymph node dissection (lymph positive) | - Elderly<br>- Worst prognosis<br>- Palliative treatment: radiation therapy chemotherapy (doxorubicin + platin) surgical debulking |

**Thyroid Examination**

| Hypothyroidism | Hyperthyroidism |
|---|---|
| ▪ **Hashimoto's thyroiditis:**<br>  - Female<br>  - Antibody of TG+ TPO<br>  - Histology (lymphocytes)<br>  - Risk factor for thyroid Lymphoma<br>  - TSH high<br>  - T3,4 low<br><br>▪ **Treatment**<br>  - Thyroxine<br><br>▪ **Other causes:**<br>  - Following hyperthyroidism treatment (thyroidectomy, radioiodine therapy)<br>  - lithium<br>  - hypopituitary(Sheehan syndrome) | ▪ **Graves' disease**<br>  - female<br>  - TSH low<br>  - T3,4 high<br>  - radioiodine scan<br><br>▪ **Specific:**<br>  - Thyroid acropachy<br>  - Pretibial myxedema<br>  - Thyroid bruit<br>  - Graves eye diseases (eye changes)<br><br>▪ **Other causes:**<br>  - Toxic multinodular goitre<br>  - toxic adenoma<br>  - Struma ovarii<br>  - subacute or postpartum thyroiditis<br>  - TSH-producing pituitary tumor |

❖ **Treatment for Hyperthyroidism:**

1. **Medicine**
- Carbimazole
- PTU: suitable during pregnancy
- **Side effects:** agranulocytosis(if fever +WBC<1000 stop the drugs), rash, hepatotoxicity.
- Propranolol (beta blocker): for tremor and cardiac symptoms

2. **Radioiodine therapy (I 131):** Good for toxic adenoma
- **Contradictions:**
- Youth
- pregnancy
- breastfeeding
- **Side effects:**
- Hypothyroidism

3. **Thyroidectomy**
- **lump:**
a. Midline

# Thyroid Examination

- Goitre (moves up on swallowing)
- Thyroglossal cyst(remnant of the thyroglossal duct.) :moves with tongue protrusion (sistrunk is surgery )

**b. lateral:**
- Carotid artery aneurysm(pulsatile )
- Cystic hygroma
- Branchial cyst

**c. lymph nodes**, sebaceous cyst ,lipoma

- **Grading system for thyroid associated ophthalmopathy**

Pneumonic = **NO SPECS**
**N:** no signs
**O:** only sign : upper lid retraction; Dalrymple
**S:** soft tissue involvement (edema, Chemosis, lagophthalmos)
**P:** proptosis
**E:** EOM involvement
**C:** corneal involvement (SPK)
**S:** sight loss (optic nerve compression)

- **Eyes complications:**
- Steroid
- Orbital decompression

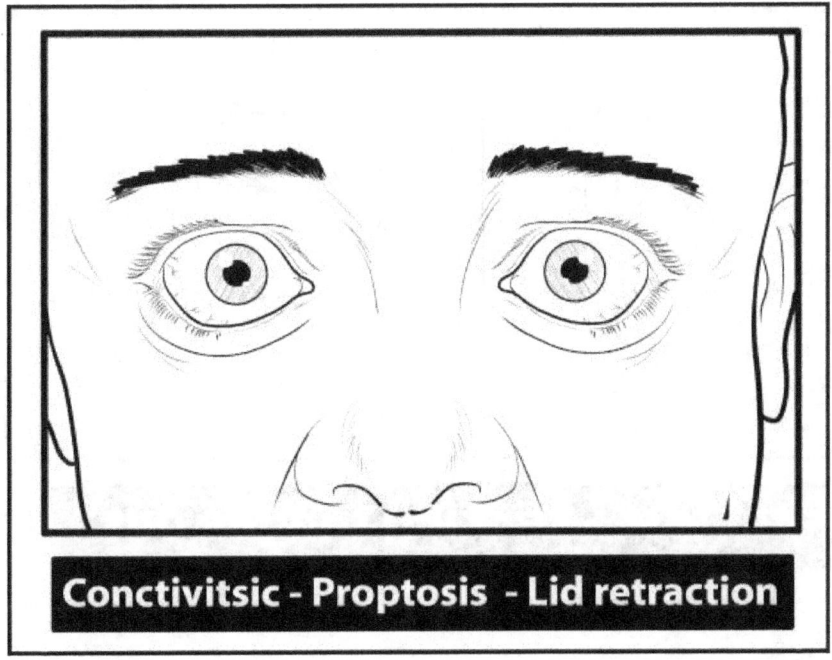
Conctivitsic - Proptosis - Lid retraction

# Thyroid Examination

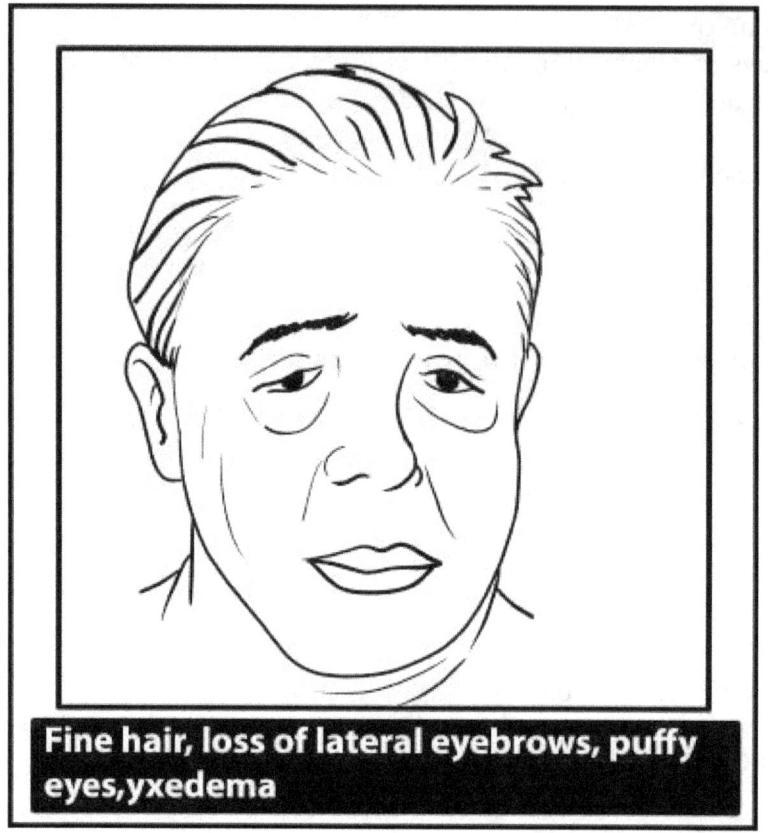

Fine hair, loss of lateral eyebrows, puffy eyes, yxedema

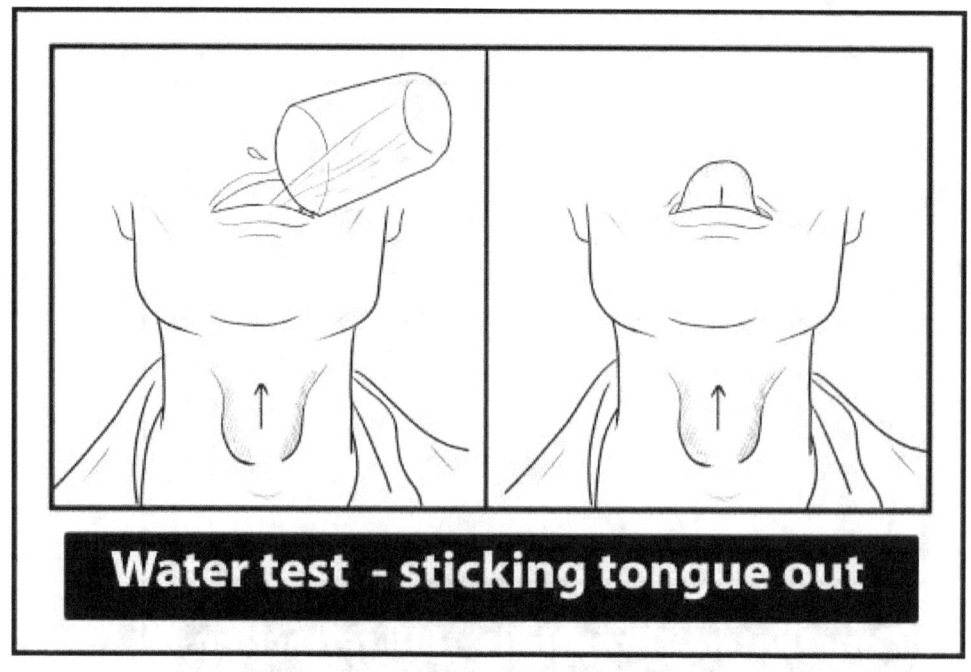

Water test - sticking tongue out

# Thyroid Examination

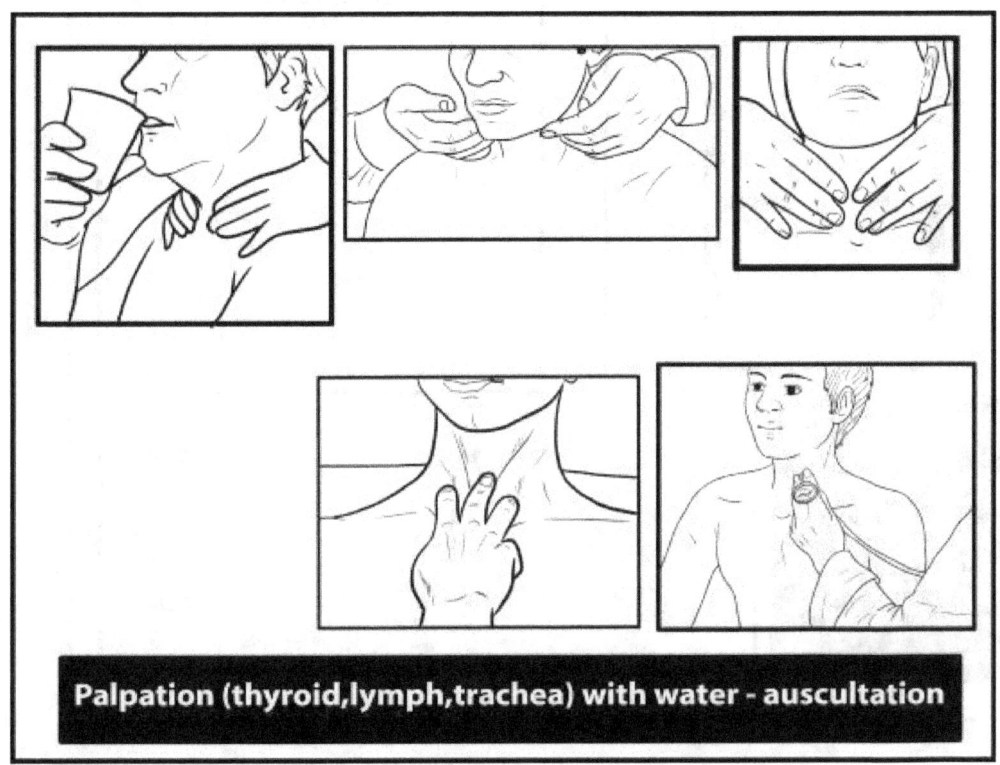

Palpation (thyroid, lymph, trachea) with water - auscultation

# Thyroid Examination

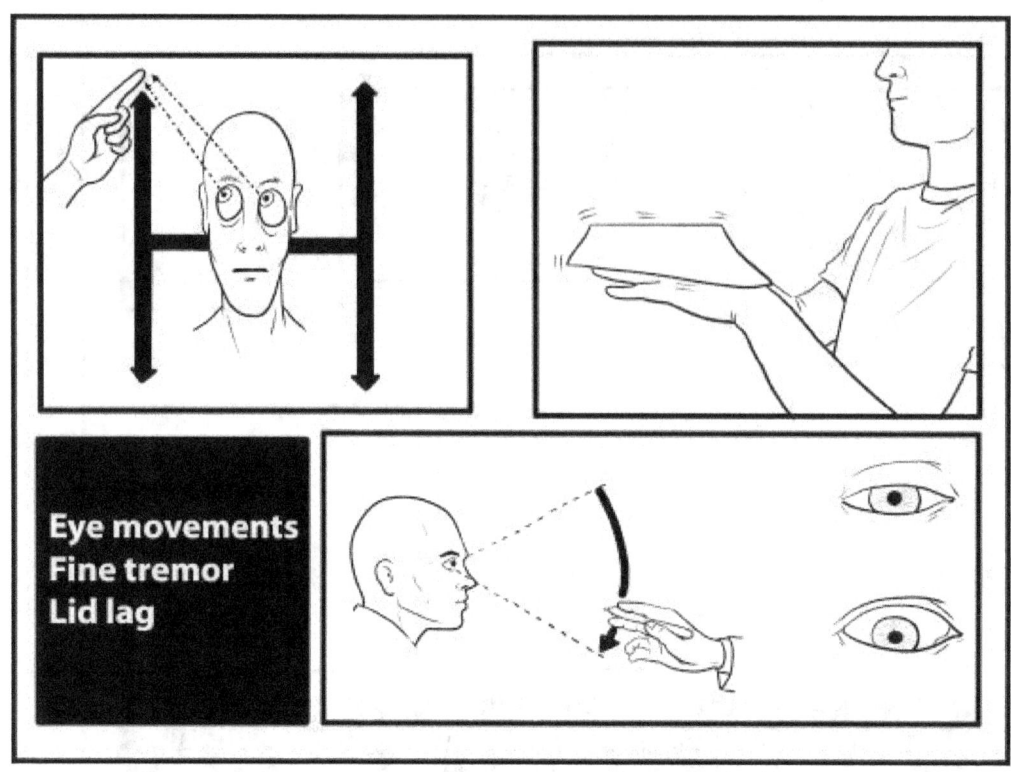

Eye movements
Fine tremor
Lid lag

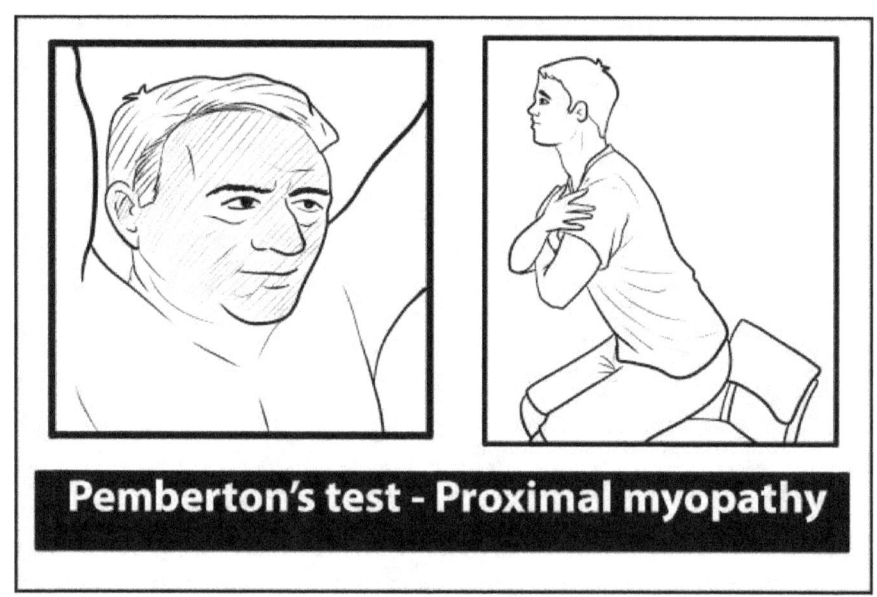

Pemberton's test - Proximal myopathy

**Thyroid Examination**

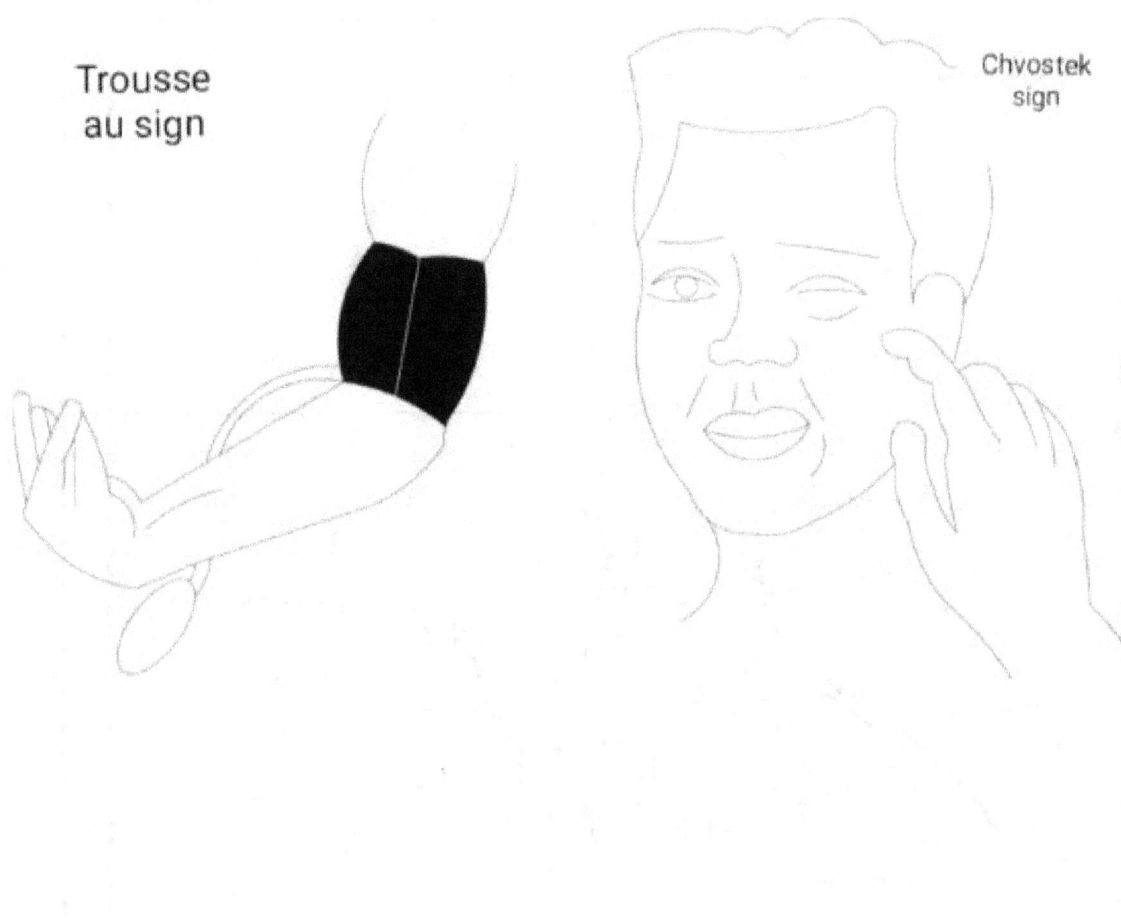

**Thyroid Examination**

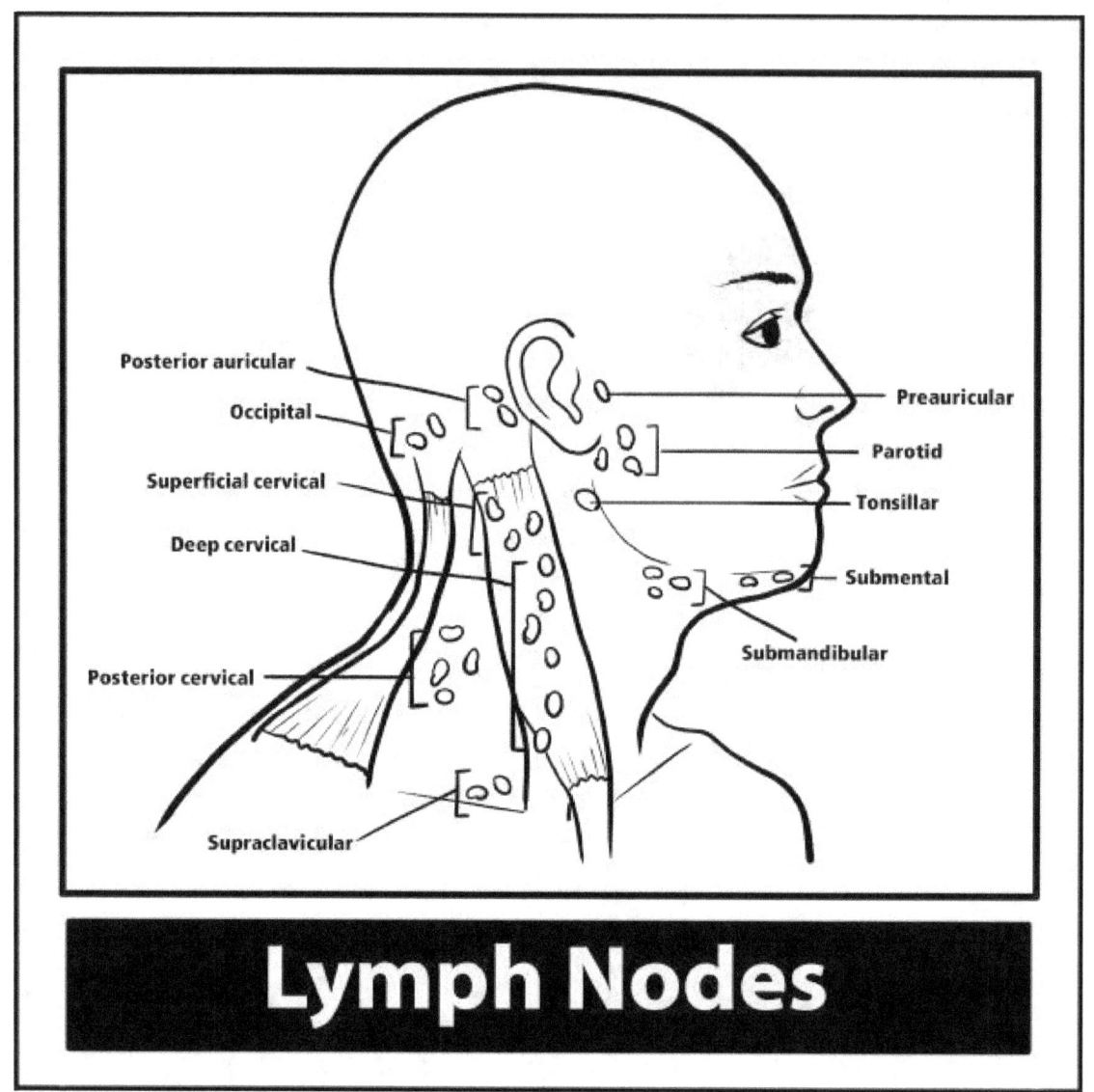

# Thyroid Examination

Borders of anterior triangle = superiorly (inferior border of mandible), laterally (anterior border of sternocleidomastoid), medially (midline of neck)
Borders of posterior triangle = posteriorly (trapezius), anteriorly (sternocleidomastoid) inferiorly (omohyoid muscle)

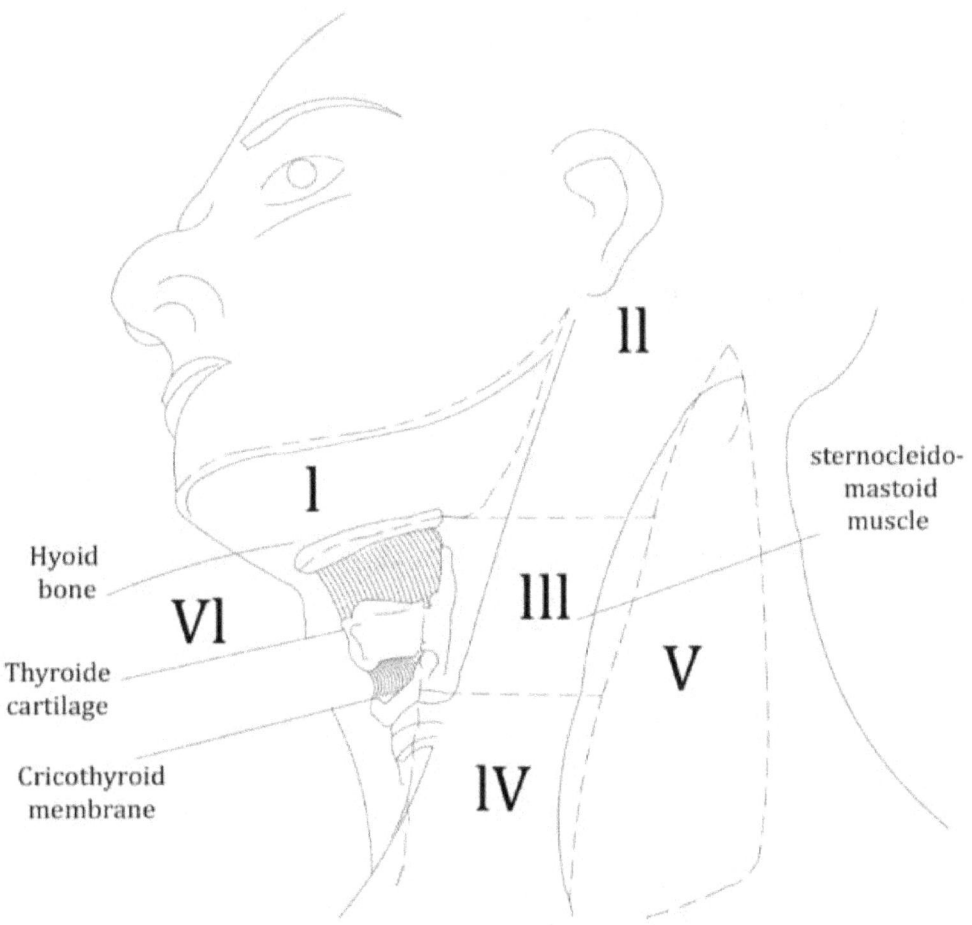

# Thyroid Examination

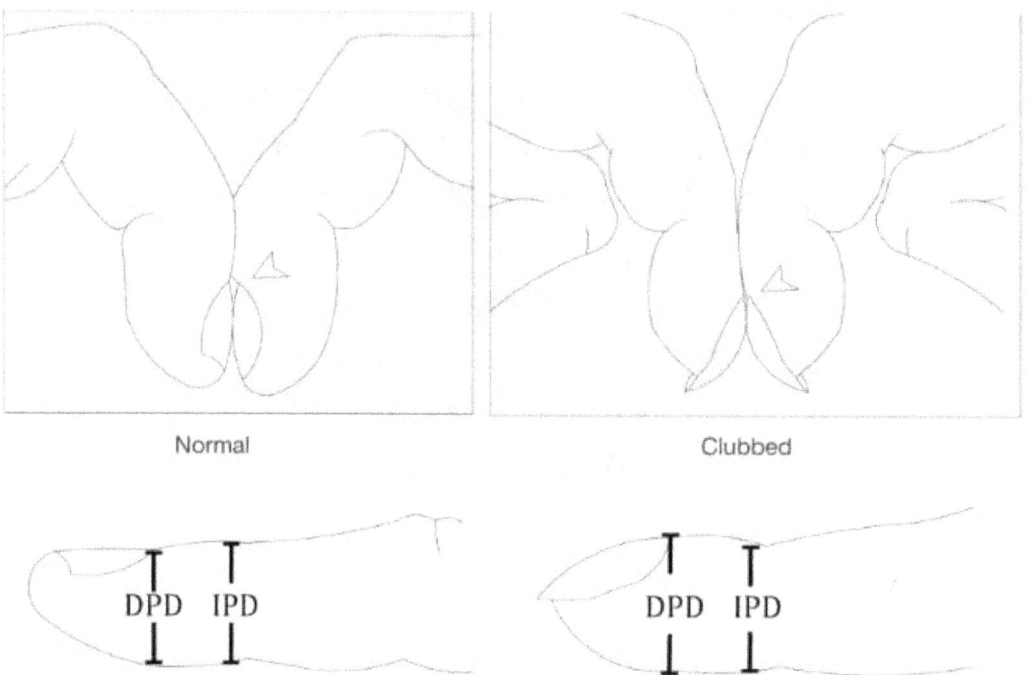

DPD : Distal phalangeal depth
IPD : Interphanalageal depth

# Cardio Examination

| | |
|---|---|
| **General** | 1. Wash hands, introduce yourself, get name and age, explain your roles and gain permission<br>2. lying in 45 degrees bed & supported by pillows, chest exposed<br>3. around bed: drug(GTN), ECG, catheter patient: cyanosis, pain, (comment on number of pillows, dyspnea, cardiac cachexia (CHF))<br>4. Obvious features of turner syndrome(bicuspid aortic valve), marfan syndrome(AR), ankylosing spondylitis (AR) |
| **Inspection** | 1. **Hands**:<br>• Digital Clubbing (IE, atrial myxoma, congenital heart disease)<br><br>- Look from side comment on: angle between nail bed & finger(positive if loss) +anteroposterior (AP) dimension between DIP& where skin join nail (positive if the DIP is smaller)<br>- Schamroth sign<br><br>• Peripheral cyanosis<br>• Splinter haemorrhages :linear haemorrhages(IE)<br>• Tar stains (smoker)<br>• temperature: cold (CHF)<br>• tendon xanthomata (hyperlipidemia)<br>• Osler's nodes(IE)painful fingers(Out in fingers)<br>• Janeway lesions(IE)painless (thenar, hypothenar)<br>• Capillary(nail) refill time: longer than 2-3 sec (abnormal)<br>• Koilonychia (anemia cause angina &SOB)<br><br>2. **Arm**:<br>• **Radial pulse**:<br>a) **Rate**: Bradycardia <60 bpm; tachycardia >100 bpm.<br>b) **Rhythm**: regular or irregular<br>*atrial fibrillation irregularly irregular pulse<br><br>c) **Volume, Character** (better at carotid)<br>• Water hammer pulse(collapsing pulse):<br>- Rule out any pain in shoulder<br>- Wrap your fingers around Pt wrist(palmer finger sides covering the radial and ulnar artery feeling the pulse<br>- Raise patient Hand<br>- There pulses will disappear for a moment then reappear again : water hammer pulse (aortic regurgitation) |

# Cardio Examination

- Radio-radial delay: cervical rib, aortic aneurysm
- Radio-femoral delay: aortic coarctation
- BP: wide or narrow pulse pressure
  Pulse pressure is the difference between the systolic and diastolic blood pressure.

needles markings (IE)

3. **Head and neck**
- Corneal arcus and xanthelasma(hyperlipidemia)
- Pallor conjunctiva(anemia)
- Scleral icterus (Mechanical hemolysis, RHF)
- Malar flush (mitral stenosis)
- Elfin facies Williams syndrome (SVAS)
- Under tongue: central cyanosis
- Dental hygiene (IE)
- High-arched palate (marfan syndrome)
- Carotid pulse for volume, character (never both together)

4. **JVP:**
- Patient at 45 degrees with head turned to the left
- Comment :
- Visible + not palpable + decrease with inspiration + filled from above if pressure is applied
- Using ruler to measure the distance between upper pulsatile point in vein and sternal angle
- Abnormal > 4 cm
- Hepatojugular reflux: apply pressure on the liver for 20 second, JVP will rise
- **Causes of raised JVP:**

a. Heart:
- RHF, tricuspid regurgitation

b. Pulmonary:
- PE, COPD (cor pulmonale)

c. Other:
- SVC obstruction (lung cancer)
- Beck's triad (cardiac tamponade) 3 D's:

Distant heart sounds

Distended jugular veins

Decreased arterial pressure

# Cardio Examination

|  |  |
|---|---|
| | **5. Chest** <br> • Pectus excavatum (funnel chest) <br> • Pectus carinatum (pigeon chest) <br> • Scars: <br> a. Midline sternotomy scar: <br> - CABG: with leg(saphenous) or arm(radial) scar (vein harvesting) <br> - valve replacement <br> b. Left submammary thoracotomy scar: mitral valvotomy. <br> c. Infraclavicular **scars with bulge:** pacemaker or defibrillator implantation scars. <br> • visible pulsations (apex beat) |
| **Palpation** | a. **Apex beat**: midclavicular line, 5th ICS <br> ∗ if difficult to feel ask to roll to left <br> b. pressure overload due AS or HTN: <br> (heaving) forceful and sustained impulse. <br> - volume loaded (thrusting) due MR ,dilated cardiomyopathy= displaced non-sustained impulse. <br> - **Impalpable apex beat**: overweight, hyperinflated lung (asthma, emphysema), dextrocardia <br> - **Displaced**: left ventricular dilatation, AR,MR HTN, dilated cardiomyopathy, chest deformities <br> c. **Heaves:** right ventricular hypertrophy or dilatation (pulmonary hypertension) <br> d. **Thrills**: murmurs |
| **Auscultation:** <br><br> ▪ **Lub-dub** <br> • **1st sound:** closure of mitral and tricuspid <br> • **2nd sounds:** Closure of aortic and pulmonary <br><br> ▪ **S1-systole-S2-diastole** | • listen with both diaphragm and bell: <br> a) 5th ICS in midclavicular line: mitral valve <br> b) left LSB, 4 or 5th ICS: tricuspid valve <br> c) left sternal edge,2nd ICS: pulmonary valve <br> d) right sternal edge, 2nd intercostal space: aortic valve <br> • maneuvers: increase sound of murmur <br> a) mitral stenosis(bell) <br> - Ask patient to turn into their left side <br> - auscultate mitral valve <br> - Take a deep breath in and out using mouth and hold your breath at the end of expiration <br> b) aortic regurgitation (diaphragm) <br> - Ask patient to sit upright <br> - auscultate at LSB <br> - Take a deep breath in and out using mouth and hold your breath at the end of expiration <br> ▪ Other: |

## Cardio Examination

| | |
|---|---|
| While your hand on carotid artery: pulsation indicates systole stage<br><br>• bell for 3rd ,4th sounds, low pitch<br>• diaphragm for high pitch sounds | - auscultate carotid artery bruits: hold bell over carotid artery and ask patient to breathe in and out and then hold it<br>• **any murmur heard:**<br>- Timing<br>a. systole: AS ,MR ,VSD ,HOCM ,pulmonary stenosis<br>b. diastole: AR,MS<br>- Location (valve)<br>- radiation: radiation to axilla (mitral regurgitation), radiation to the carotids (aortic stenosis)<br>- character (harsh, blowing, rumbling, low or high pitched)<br>- Grades<br>- Prosthetic heart valve<br>- Murmur changes with breathing:<br>a. Louder on inspiration=right-sided valves(tricuspid ,pulmonary)<br>b. Louder with expiration= left sided valves (mitral , aortic)<br>▪ **Extra sounds:**<br>a) **3rd heart sound:**<br>- Volume overload<br>- Not pathological in young adult<br>- LVF (if with tachycardia gallop rhythms)<br>- Mitral or aortic Regurgitation<br>- Myocardial infarction<br>b) **4th heart sound:**<br>- Pressure overload<br>- LV Hypertrophy<br>- Aortic stenosis<br>- HOCM<br>▪ **Murmur Grades:**<br>• **Grade 1:** only expert<br>• **Grade 2:** quiet, soft<br>• **Grade 3:** loud, no thrill<br>• **Grade 4:** loud murmur, with a thrill<br>• **Grade 5**: Very loud, with thrill, heard over wide area with stethoscope partly off<br>• **Grade 6:** heard without stethoscope |
| | ▪ **RHF:**<br>• Auscultate lung bases for bibasal crepitations<br>• Palpate for pitting ankle oedema |
| **To complete** | • **Urinalysis:** Haematuria (endocarditis, vasculitis), glucose (diabetes) and protein (HTN)<br>• **Abdominal examination:** hepatomegaly(RHF), splenomegaly (IE) |

## Cardio Examination

- Peripheral vascular examination
- ECG, ABG, CXR

- **Pulsus paradoxus**: decrease in SBP >10 mmHg in inspiration
  - **Lung pathology** (COPD, Asthma, PE)
  - **Heart pathology**

| Central cyanosis | Peripheral cyanosis |
|---|---|
| • Decreased oxygen saturation | • Normal oxygen saturation |
| • Skin and mucosa(tongue ,lips)<br>• Warm hands with clubbing | • Skin (hands ,tip of nose)<br>• Cold hands |
| • Congenital right to left shunt (fallot tetralogy)<br>• Pulmonary( COPD, acute pulmonary edema<br>• IPF, pulmonary embolism) | • Heart failure<br>• PVD<br>• Cold<br>• Raynaud syndrome |

❖ **Splinter hemorrhage:**
1. IE
2. Truma
3. RA
4. Vasculitis

- **Clubbing:** grades
1. Angle between nail and nail bed loss, nail bed fluctuation
2. Parrot beak appearance
3. Drumstick appearance
4. Hypertrophic osteoarthropathy (HOA)

- **Jugular Venous Pressure:**
- Indication for right atrial pressure
- Internal jugular vein
- **Waveforms JVP**: two waves and two descent
1. A wave: right atrial contraction

# Cardio Examination

2. x descent :atrial relaxation
3. C wave: right ventricular contraction pushing tricuspid valve into right atrium
4. y descent,: tricuspid valve opening

- **Pathology:**
- Giant A wave: tricuspid valve or ventricular premature contraction
- Giant V wave a: tricuspid regurgitation
- Prominent x and y descents :constrictive heart disease.

**Indications** for CABG :

-> 70% stenosis of the proximal LAD

-Symptomatic 3-vessel disease

**Grafts types**

-Internal thoracic artery (internal mammary artery)

-Radial artery

-Great saphenous vein(mostly)

- **Tachycardia:**
1. Sinus tachycardia
2. Atrial flutter
3. Afib :Causes:
- Hyperthyroidism ,pneumonia , ischemic heart disease ,PE , pheochromocytoma

|  | Mitral Stenosis | Mitral Regurgitation |
|---|---|---|
| **Risk factors** | - **RHD(female)**<br>- Other:<br>• Congenital<br>• Lutembacher syndrome(MS+L to R shunt(ASD))<br>• Replaced valve<br>• Age( calcification )<br>• myxoma | 1. RHD<br>2. Mitral valve prolapse<br>3. IE<br>4. MI(Papillary muscle rupture)<br>5. Chordae tendineae rupture<br>6. cardiomyopathy(dilation of LV) |
| **Clinical features** | • Asymptomatic,<br>• Dyspnea on exertion<br>• Afib | • Asymptomatic<br>• Palpitation |

# Cardio Examination

| | | |
|---|---|---|
| | • Hemoptysis<br>• Pulmonary HTN (RHF, bronchitis)<br>• Malar flush | • RHF(increased JVP) symptoms |
| **Findings** | • S1 loud<br>• Opening snap followed by diastolic rumble Low-pitched murmur<br>* the nearer the opening snap to S2 (severity)<br>• Graham Steell murmur : in pulmonary HTN due MS<br>• Severe MS results when the MV opening is reduced to less than 1.5 cm2 | • Blowing, high pitched pansystolic murmur radiates to the axilla<br>• laterally displaced PMI;<br>• AFib |
| **Treatment** | ▪ **Wilkins score**<br>• AFib: warfarin<br>• Diuretic for CHF<br>• Antiarrhythmic drug :digoxin<br><br>Usually repaired not replaced<br><br>▪ **Indication for valvotomy:**<br>- severe +symptomatic<br>• Percutaneous balloon valvuloplasty<br>• Valvotomy(widening the valve)<br>• Valve replacement: indicated for<br>- If severe +symptomatic+ Left atrial thrombosis<br><br>OR<br><br>- moderated/severe MR | ▪ antiarrhythmic drug :digoxin<br>▪ **Indication**:<br>• symptomatic patients with severe MR<br>• MV repair better than replacement<br>• Valve replacement Indication: Symptom |

| Aortic stenosis | Aortic regurgitation |
|---|---|

## Cardio Examination

| | |
|---|---|
| - **Congenital:** bicuspid valve (younger age)<br>- Calcified aortic stenosi(elderly)<br>- **Other:** Rheumatic fever, Idiopathic hypertrophic subaortic stenosis, HOCM | - Marfan syndrome<br>- aortic dissection(acute )<br>- infective endocarditis, syphilitic aortitis<br>- **Other:** ankylosing spondylitis ,HTN ,Rheumatic fever |
| - Progressive dyspnea, angina, syncope on exertion | - Dyspnea, fatigue on exertional<br>- Left heart failure symptoms<br>- Palpitation |
| - **Ejection click:** early systolic harsh murmur<br>- Radiate to neck (carotid)<br>- The more severe the stenosis, the nearer the murmur peak to s2<br>- low pulse pressure<br><br>- pulses parvus et tardus: reduced in amplitude and rises slowly to its peak<br>- Soft S2<br>- S4<br>- Heaving non-displaced Apex beat.<br>- Angiodysplasia (lower GI bleeding)<br>- Systolic thrill<br><br>- Severe AS :<br>- Transvalvular jet velocity≥4 m/s<br>- Mean valve gradient of ≥40 mm Hg.<br>- Valve area <1 cm | - **Early Diastolic:** blowing decrescendo high pitched.<br>- Wide pulse pressure<br>- Water hammer pulse<br>- Austin Flint murmur<br>- **Signs:**<br>- **De Musset:** nodding of the head at the same time of pulse.<br>- **Corrigan:** carotid pulsation visible at neck.<br>- Quincke's sign Capillary pulsations on nails<br>- **Traube:** pistol shot systolic sound over femoral artery.<br>- **Duroziez's sign:** systolic & diastolic murmur over the femoral artery when applying pressure on femoral artery<br>- Austin Flint murmur: low-pitched diastolic rumble<br>- **Hill's sign:** The difference between systolic BP in lower limb & Upper limb > 60 mmHg.<br>- Müller sign: Uvula bobs |
| 1. Valve replacement(best)<br>2. Transcatheter AVR(unfit for surgery)<br>3. balloon valvuloplasty<br><br>- **Indications for replacement:**<br>- Symptomatic<br>- severe AS | 1. **Valve replacement Indications:**<br><br>- acute presentation<br>- symptomatic<br>- undergoing cardiac surgery |

## Cardio Examination

| - moderate/Severe AS + undergoing heart or aorta surgery (CABG, surgery on aorta, | |
|---|---|

Examples of **Systolic** murmurs :

1. **Aortic sclerosis**
   a. Systolic murmur similar to AS but does not radiate and normal pulse volume (without pulsus parvus et tardus)

   a. Pulmonary stenosis
   b. Hypertrophic obstructive cardiomyopathy(HOCM)
   c. Supravalvular aortic stenosis (williams syndrome).

### ❖ Prosthetic Heart Valves:

- **Types:**

| Types | Mechanical | Bioprosthetic |
|---|---|---|
| • Lifespan | • Longer for 30 years | • Shorter for about 15 years<br>* needs reoperation |
| • anti-clotting | • Lifelong(warfarin) | • For the first few months |
|  | • younger<br>• long life expectancy | • Good for who wish to be pregnant in the future due to warfarin (teratogenic) and short life expectancy |
|  |  | • Hard to distinguish between it and normal heart valve by stethoscope |

- **Complication:**
  - Structural Valve failure
  - IE
  - Paravalvular leak
  - Degeneration
  - Thrombosis
  - Mismatch valve (too small)
  - Mechanical haemolysis

## Cardio Examination

| Aortic valve prostheses | Mitral valve prostheses |
|---|---|
| -location : 2 ICS<br><br>- heart sound(HS) :<br><br>   a. Normal first HS<br>   b. Metallic second HS<br><br>*Systolic murmur is normal but diastolic is not | -Location : apex<br>- heart sound(HS) :<br>   c. metallic first HS<br>   d. normal second HS |

❖ **Myocardial infarction:**
- Transmural infarction (ST elevation)
- Subendocardial infarction (Non ST elevation)
- troponin (sensitive and specific)

❖ **Heart failure:**
- **Causes**
  - MI, myocarditis, cardiomyopathy, Mitral stenosis, atrial Myxoma
  - Valves disorders, TN
* High output HF: anemia, AV, hyperthyroidism

- **Clinical Features:**
  ➢ **Left heart failure:**
  - [POD: PND, Orthopnea, dyspnea on exertion
  - Pinky forty sputum
  - Oliguria, peripheral cyanosis, fatigue

  ➢ **Right heart failure:**
  - Congested neck vein (JVP)
  - Bilateral leg swelling
  - Enlarged tender liver
* **Staging by NYHA:** severity of the heart failure with types of physical Activity

- **X-ray ABCDE:**
- Alveolar oedema (bat's wings)

**Cardio Examination**

- Kerley B lines (interstitial oedema)
- Cardiomegaly
- Dilated prominent upper lobe vessels
- Effusion (pleural)

- **Echo:**
- **Systolic dysfunction**=Low ejection fraction (low)
- **Diastolic dysfunction** = normal EF

- **Tricuspid Regurgitation:**
- Due to Right heart dilation from:
- Left heart failure
- Inferior wall MI
- Cor pulmonale (pulmonary pathology like COPD)
- Tricuspid endocarditis (IV drug).

- **Clinical features:**
- RHF (JVP, hepatomegaly ascites, edema)
- Pulsatile liver
- Holosystolic murmur
- Prominent V

❖ **Rheumatic Heart Disease:**
- Streptococcal pharyngitis
- Mitral valve (stenosis)

- **Infective Endocarditis:**

- S. aureus
- Streptococcus viridans
- Prosthetic valve endocarditis((S. epidermidis)
- Duke criteria
- fever +murmur(new)
- Splenomegaly
- clubbing
- Janeway and Osler nodes
- Roth spot

## Cardio Examination

| | Major Criteria | | Minor Criteria |
|---|---|---|---|
| J | Joint Involvement | C | CRP Increased |
| O | O looks like a heart = myocarditis | A | Arthralgia |
| N | Nodules , subcutaneous | F | Fever |
| E | Erythema marginatum | E | Elevated ESR |
| S | Sydenham chorea | P | Prolonged PR Interval |
| | | A | Anamnesis of Rheumatism |
| | | L | Leukocytosis |

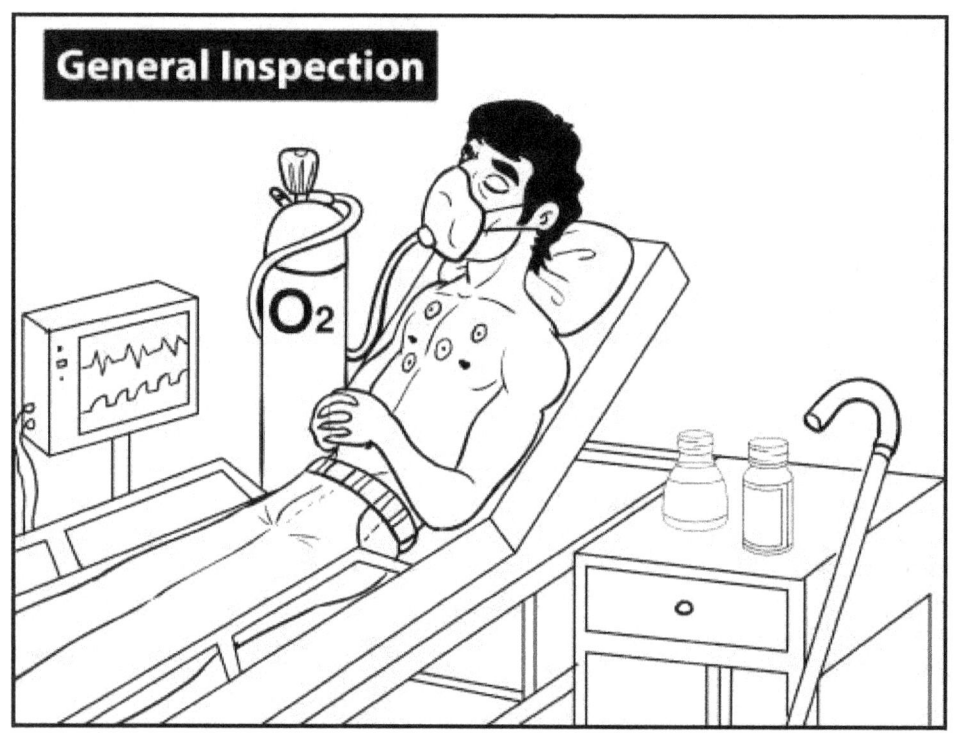

42

**Cardio Examination**

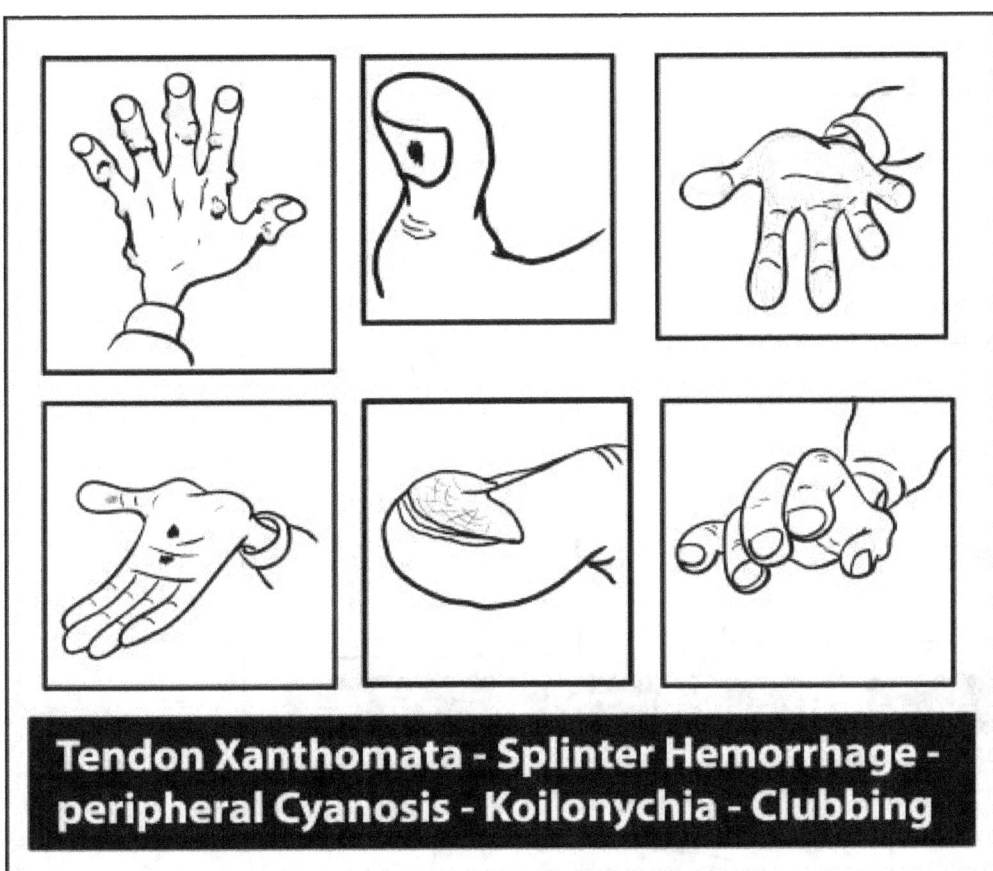

Tendon Xanthomata - Splinter Hemorrhage - peripheral Cyanosis - Koilonychia - Clubbing

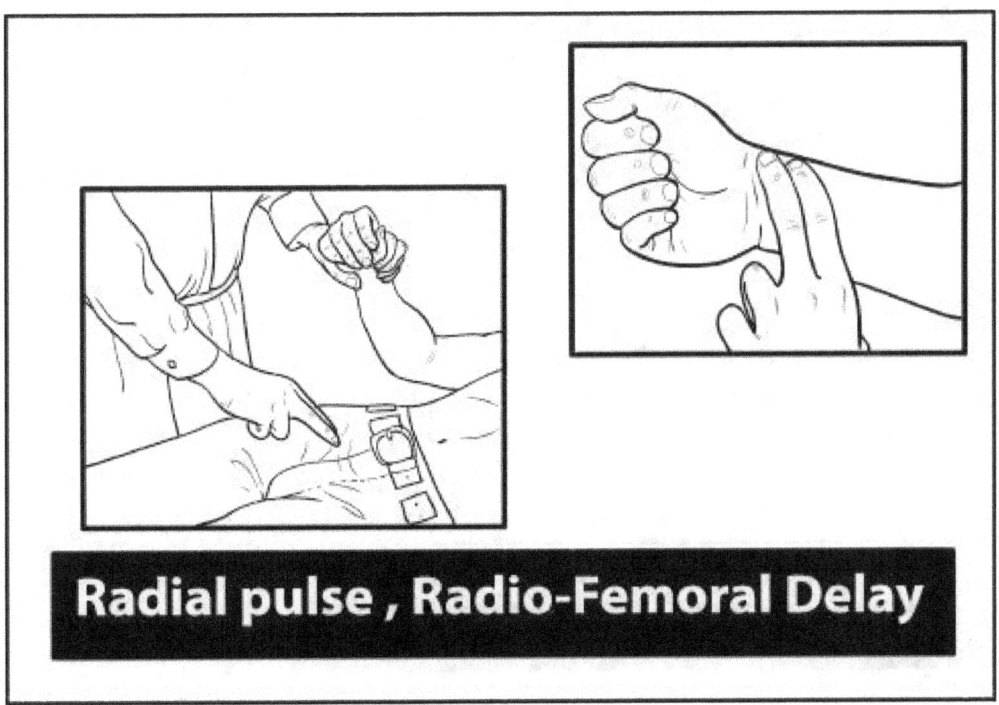

Radial pulse, Radio-Femoral Delay

## Cardio Examination

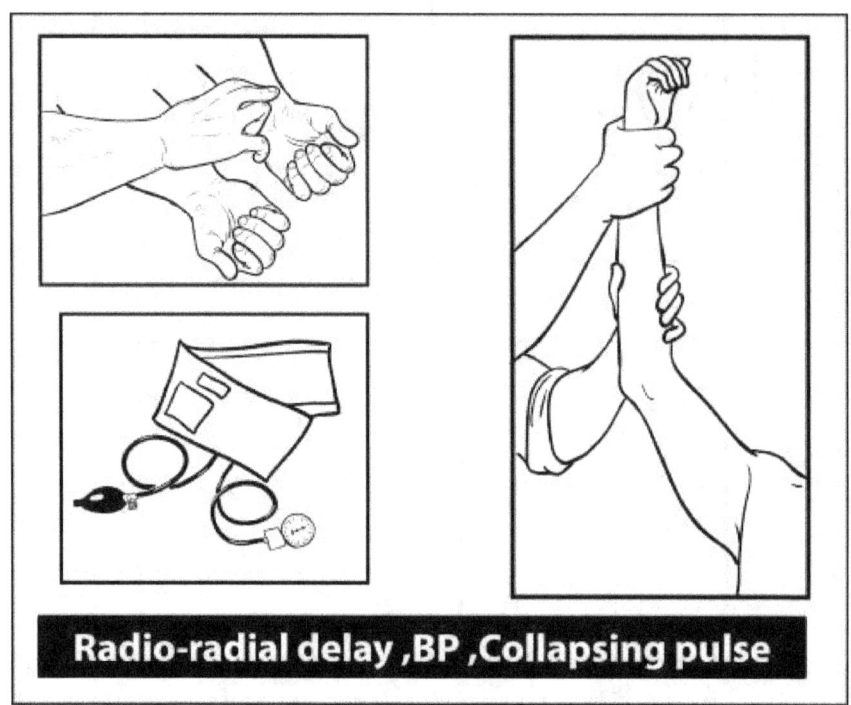

Radio-radial delay, BP, Collapsing pulse

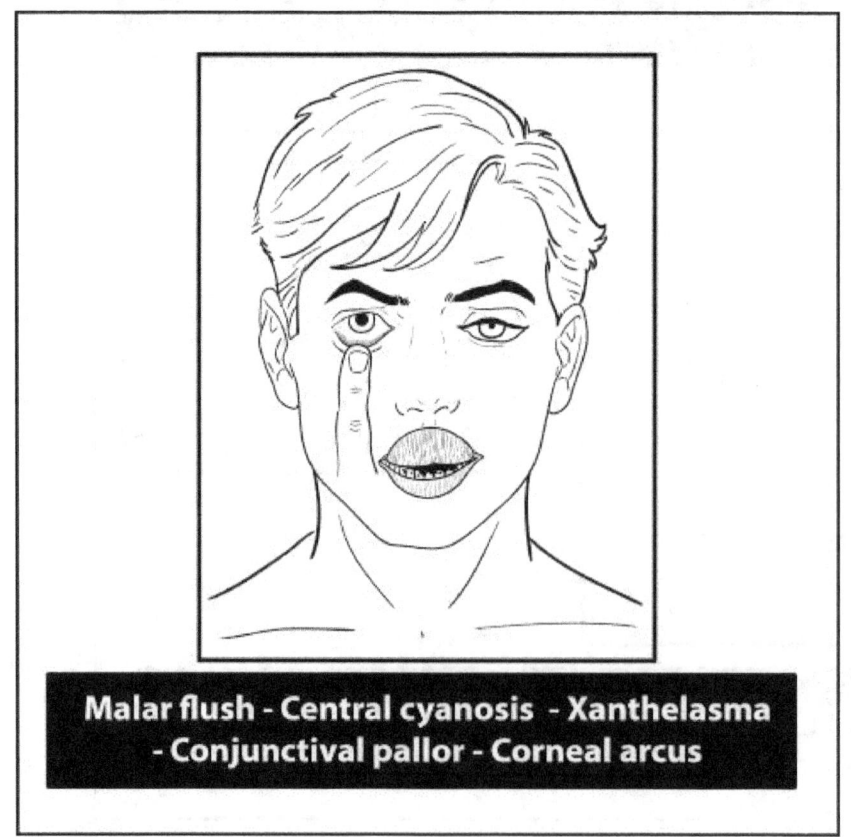

Malar flush - Central cyanosis - Xanthelasma - Conjunctival pallor - Corneal arcus

# Cardio Examination

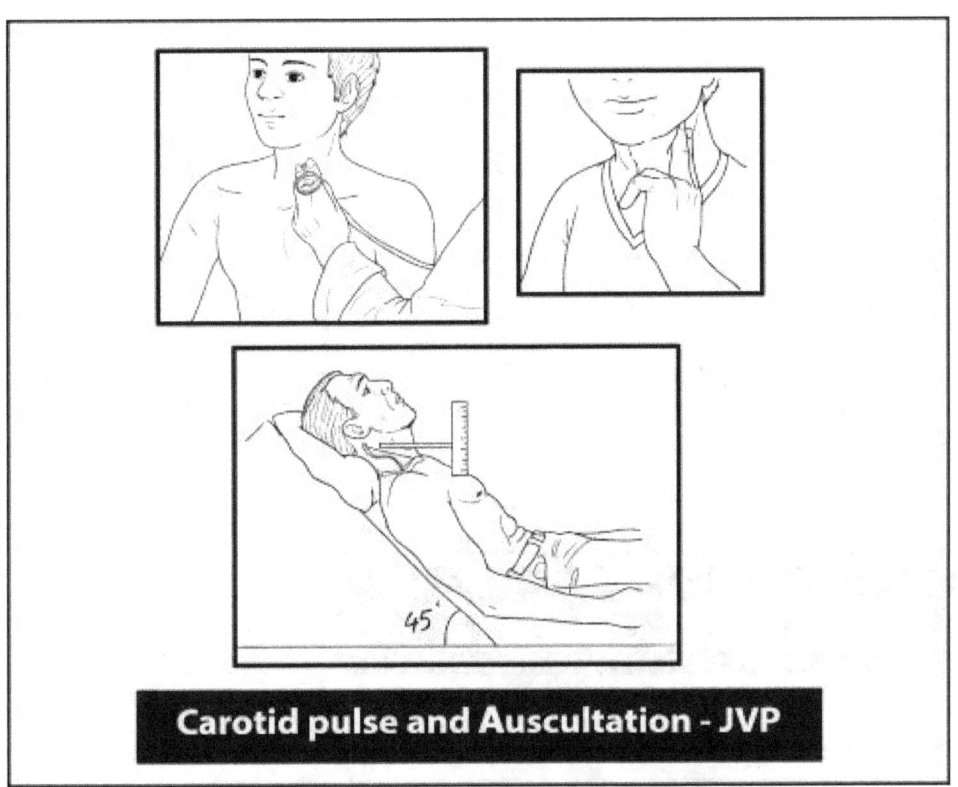

**Carotid pulse and Auscultation - JVP**

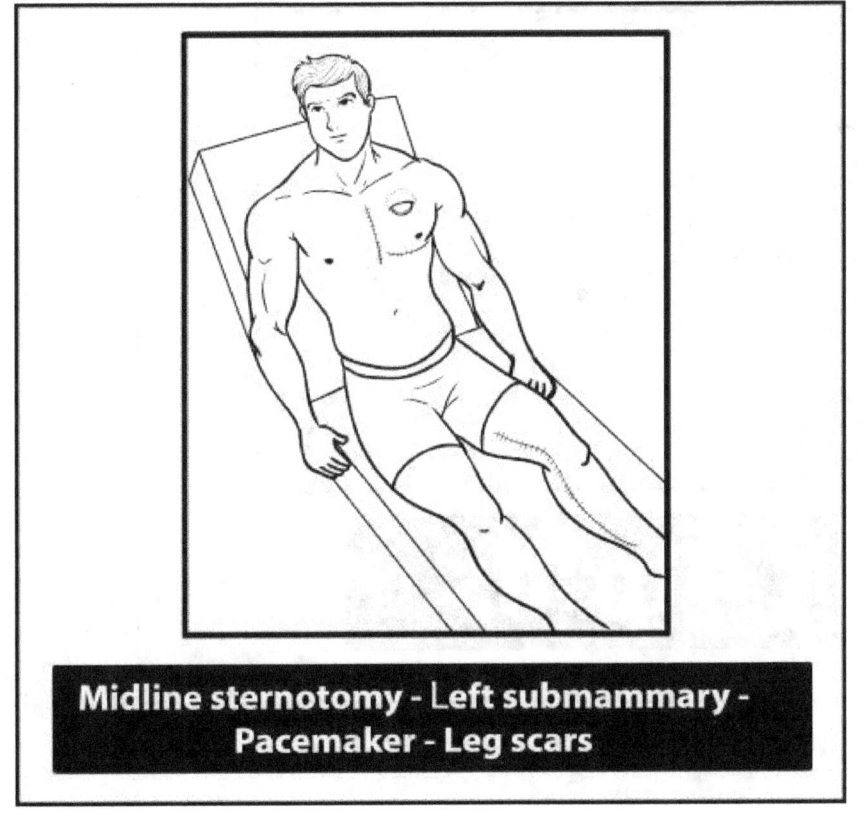

**Midline sternotomy - Left submammary - Pacemaker - Leg scars**

# Cardio Examination

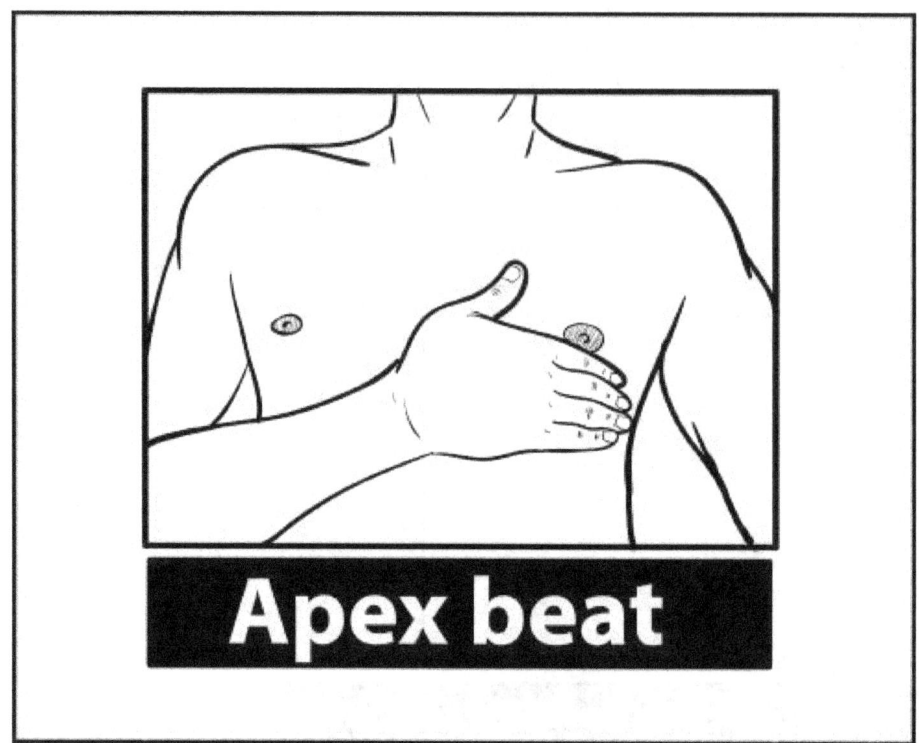

Apex beat

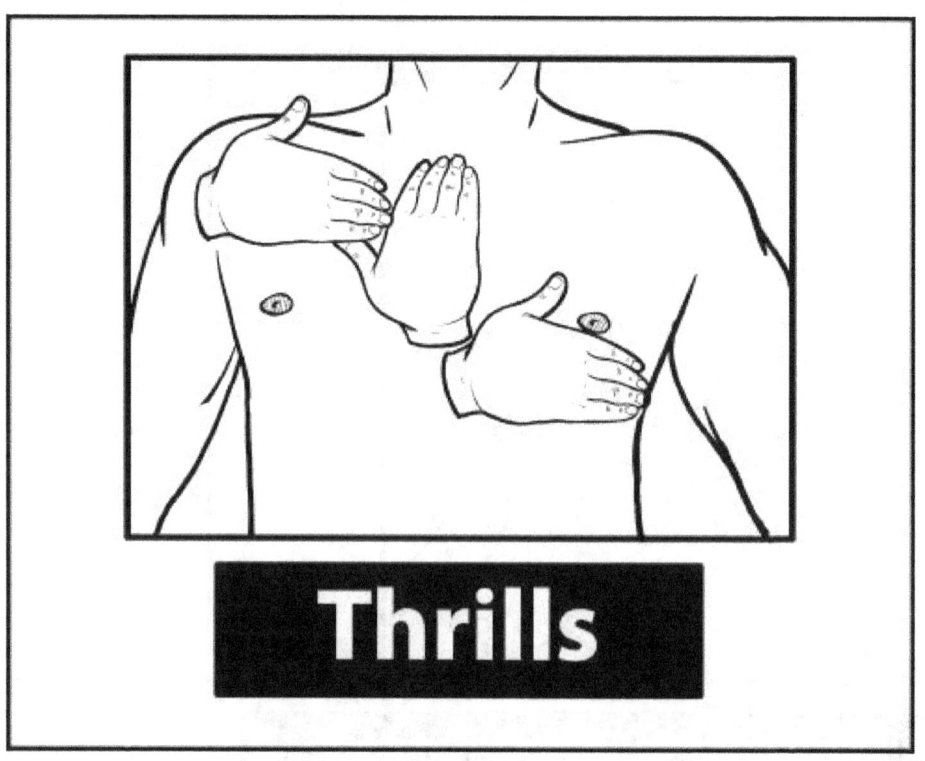

Thrills

# Cardio Examination

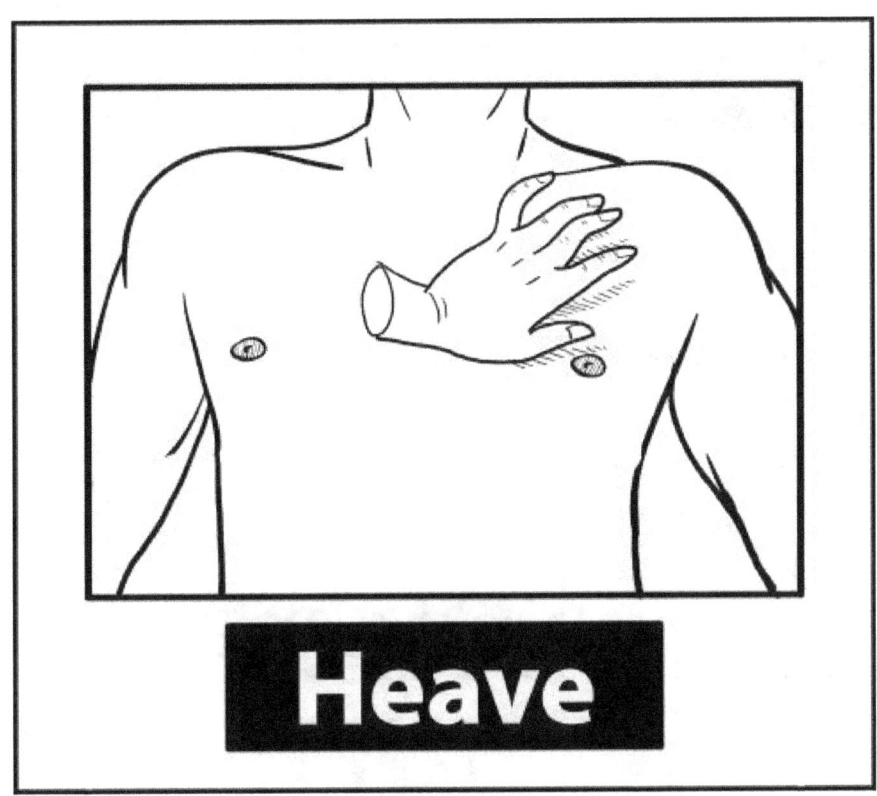

**Heave**

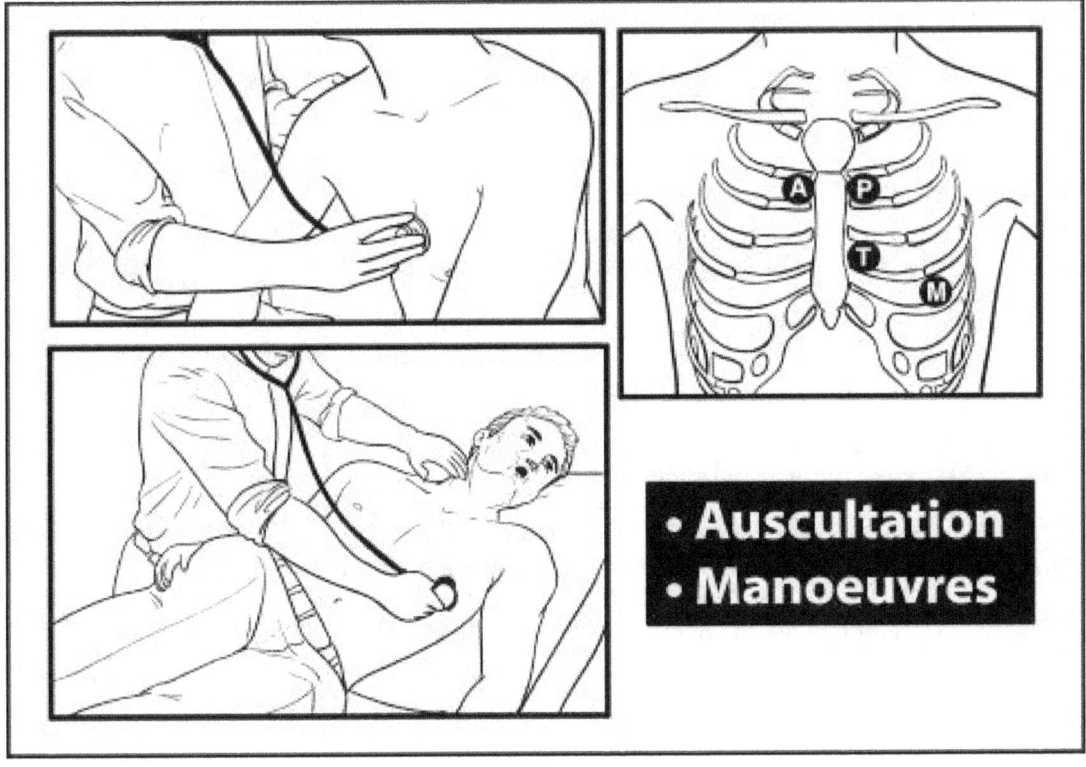

- **Auscultation**
- **Manoeuvres**

# Cardio Examination

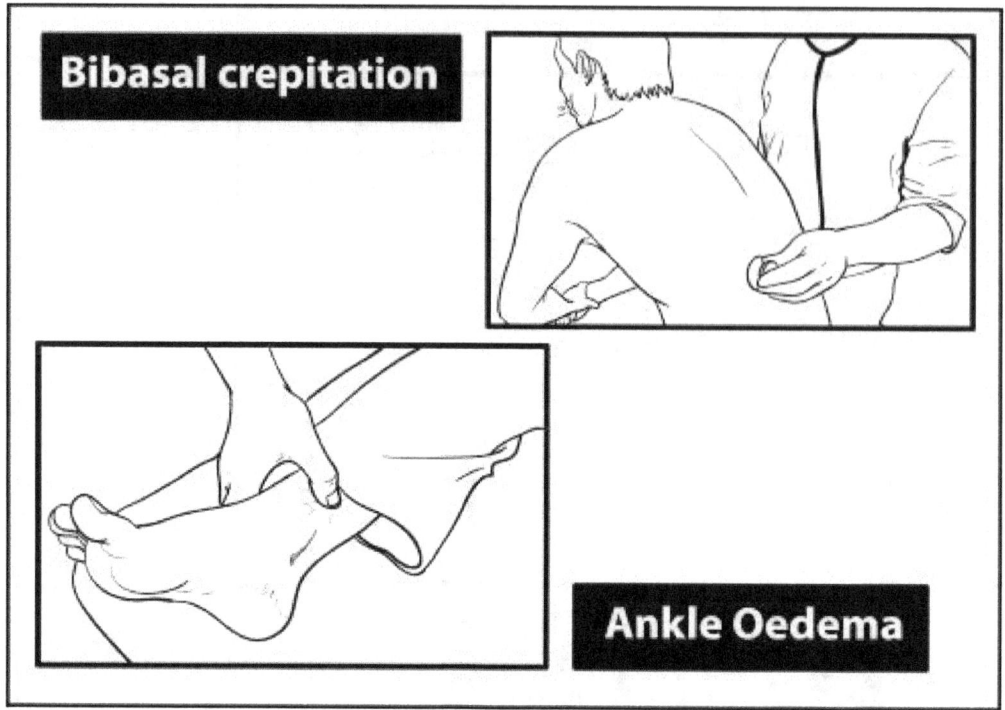

a-c-v waves
x - y descents

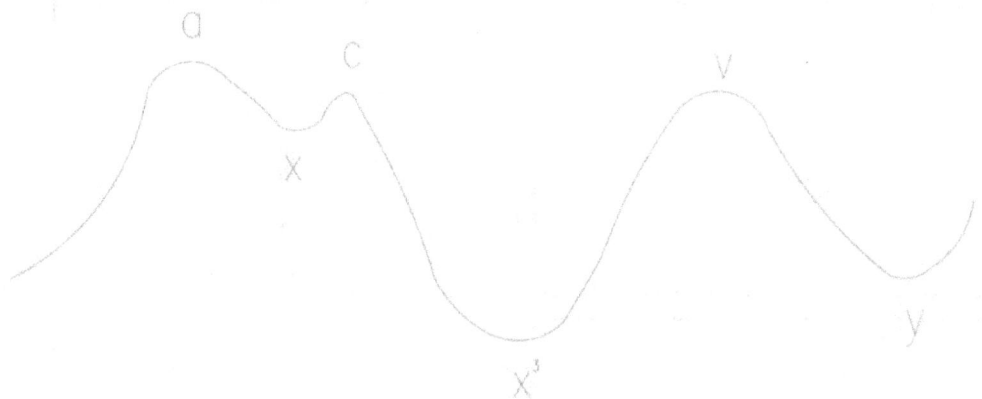

a- atrial contraction
x- atrial relaxation
c- bulging of tricuspid valve with ventricular contraction
$x_3$-downward movement of tricuspid valve with ventricular contraction
v-passive atrial filling
y- atrial emptying with opening of the tricuspid valve

# Respiratory Examination

| | |
|---|---|
| **General** | 1. Wash hands, introduce yourself, get name and age, explain your roles and gain permission<br>2. Lying in 45 degrees bed, chest exposed<br>3. Around bed: ventilation machines(BiPAP), peak flow meter, sputum bag, inhalers, oxygen masks<br>4. Patient: cyanosis, cachexia(emphysema), dyspnea, distress, cough, noise (stridor, wheeze), use of accessory muscles, pursed lips |
| **Inspection** | 1. **Hand:**<br>• **Clubbing:** Fibrosing Alveolitis, Bronchial, carcinoma, Mesothelioma, CF, bronchiectasis, lung abscess, Hypertrophic pulmonary osteoarthropathy(SCC)<br>• **Tar staining**<br>• **Temperature:** cold (CHF), hot (co2 retention)<br>• peripheral cyanosis(hypoxia)<br>• **hands muscle atrophy**: pancost (apical) tumor compressing brachial plexus<br>• fine Tremor (beta agonists such as salbutamol)<br>• **Asterixis (flapping tremor):** arms outstretched, wrists dorsiflex, fingers spread, eyes closed<br>• Carbon Dioxide retention (respiratory failure)<br>• Respiratory Rate (12 per min normal)<br>• **Radial pulse:** bounding pulse (co2 retention)<br>• **BP:** hypotension (pneumonia, tension pneumothorax), Pulsus paradoxus(asthma)<br>2. **Head and neck:**<br>• Conjunctival pallor(anemia)<br>• Horner's syndrome (apical lung tumor): miosis, ptosis, anhidrosis<br>• Use light torch to examine nose (nasal polyps and aspirin sensitivity)<br>• Moon face: Cushing syndrome (corticosteroid)<br>• Tongue: central cyanosis (lung diseases)<br>• JVP: Increased due RHF (cor pulmonale)<br>• Lymph node palpation<br>• Trachea<br>  a. palpate by using your three middle finger (midline or deviated)<br>  b. tracheal tug (hyperinflated lung like COPD)<br>3. **Chest:**<br>• Asymmetrical expansion<br>• **Deformities**: increase the work required to breath<br>  - Pectus Excavatum<br>  - Pectus Carinatum(asthma)<br>  - Scoliosis |

## Respiratory Examination

| | |
|---|---|
| | - Scars (chest drains in mid axillary line, lobectomy, pneumonectomy<br>- AP overexpansion (COPD)<br>- Peg tube (CF)<br>- Portacath(CF) |
| **Palpation** | - Apex beat<br>- Heave: RV hypertrophy<br>- Chest expansion: in two location<br>  - Deep breath by mouth<br>  - Reduced expansion:<br>    a. Unilateral(PPP): pleural effusion, pneumonia, pneumothorax<br>    b. Bilateral: COPD, pulmonary fibrosis<br>- Tactile fremitus:<br>Say 99 while edges on your hand placed over chest<br>  - Decreased: COPD, or pleural effusion, pneumothorax<br>  - Increased: consolidation (pneumonia) |
| **Percussion** | - Percuss the posterior thorax while patient crossing arms and both hands rested on shoulder (hug yourself)<br>- Start over supraclavicular fossa, both sides and axilla<br>- **Resonance:** normal<br>- **Dullness (fluid or solid):** pneumonia, pleural effusion, hemothorax, empyema, Fibrosis, tumor.<br>- Hyperresonance (COPD, pneumothorax, bullae) |
| **Auscultation** | - **Diaphragm**<br>  - Deep breath by mouth<br>  - Start over supraclavicular fossa, both sides and axilla<br>- **Quality of breath sounds:**<br>- **Intensity:** low in any lung pathologies<br>- **Character**:<br>  a. **Vesicular(normal):** soft, Inspiration >Expiration and no pause in between.<br>  b. **Bronchial(abnormal):** harsh Expiration>Inspiration and pause in between due fluid-filled or solid lung tissue<br>- **added sounds:**<br>  a. Fine: Late inspiratory crackles (interstitial lung disease)<br>  b. Coarse crackles: early inspiratory crackle (infection, bronchitis, fluid filled)<br>  c. Wheezes: expiration (asthma, COPD)<br>    \* if crepitation disappears after coughing then its normal secretion and not pneumonia |

## Respiratory Examination

| | |
|---|---|
| **Vocal Resonance** | • Whisper 99 and auscultate<br>- Increased (consolidation)<br>- Decreased (pleural effusion or pneumothorax) |
| **The End** | • Sputum pot<br>• O2 saturation<br>• Ankle oedema (cor pulmonale)<br>• PEFR<br>• X-ray |

❖ **Tracheal Shift:**
- **Toward the problem:**
- Pneumonectomy, Atelectasis, Pleural fibrosis
- **Away from problem:**
- Tension pneumothorax, Pleural effusion, mass(tumor)

❖ **Pancoast Tumor:**
• Apex lung tumor

- **Clinical features:**
- Horner syndrome
- C8 to T2 compression
- Wasting and weakness of the small muscles of the hand
- Radiating shoulder pain

- **Signs of respiratory distress:**
- Increased RR
- Use of accessory muscles
- Pursed lip breathing
- Cannot speak in sentence
- Pulsus paradoxus

- **Signs of CO2 Retention**
- Flapping tremor, confusion, tachypnoea, drowsiness, Chemosis
- Cyanosis, tachycardia
- Thoracotomy scar :(pneumonectomy or lobectomy)

- **Indications:**
- Lung cancer
- TB/aspergilloma

## Respiratory Examination

- Bronchiectasis
- **Finding in pneumonectomy:**
- Reduced chest expansion
- DUL
- Tracheal shift toward the resected site

- **lobectomy:**
- Only scar without any finding

- **CURB-65 Score for Pneumonia Severity:**
- Confusion
- BUN > 7 mmol/L
- Respiratory Rate ≥ 30
- SBP < 90 mmHg or DBP ≤ 60 mmHg
- Age ≥ 65

❖ **Pulmonary Function Tests:**

| | Obstruction | restricted |
|---|---|---|
| **Obstruction** | • COPD<br>• asthma | • restricted |
| **FEV1/FVC** | • <0.7<br>• *FEV1 ≥12% or ≥200 mL increases after bronchodilator = reversible airway obstruction(asthma) | • >0.7 |
| **TLC and RV** | • Increased | • Reduced |
| **DLCO** | • Increased in asthma,<br>• Reduced in COPD | • low in intrathoracic disease (Pulmonary fibrosis)<br>• Normal in extrathoracic causes(obesity, kyphosis, GBS, MG) |

❖ **Asthma**

## Respiratory Examination

- **Clinical features:**
- Young age
- Chronic episodic or continuous wheezing, dyspnea, chest tightness, cough
- Worse at night
- Improved by bronchodilator
- nasal polyps and aspirin sensitivity
- Associated with eczema, atopic dermatitis

- **Investigations:**
- **ABG:** respiratory alkalosis, hypocarbia
- PFT(spirometry):
- Both FEV1/FVC, FEV1 low
- During attacks only
- *supplying bronchodilator increase FEV1 of 12 %
- peak expiratory flow (diurnal variation)

- **Complication**
- Pneumothorax, respiratory failure, rib fracture

- **Treatments:**
- Inhalation of
- SABA(salbutamol)
- low-dose inhaled glucocorticoid
- LABA(salmeterol)
- Oral steroid
- **Other:**
  - Omalizumab: for high IgE
  - leukotriene modifier
  - theophylline

**Acute severe asthma**

- Inability to complete a sentence in one breath

- RR >25

- HR >110 beats/min

- PEF <50%

**life-threatening asthma**

- PEF <33%

- confusion, coma

- Silent chest, cyanosis

## Respiratory Examination

-Bradycardia or hypotension.

-Normal Paco2

### ❖ COPD

- **Risk factor:** smoking

- **Clinical features:**
- Chronic productive cough for 3 months or more in at least 2 consecutive years
- Progressive Dyspnea
- Blue bloater (chronic bronchitis)
- Pink puffer (emphysema)

- **Investigations:**
- **ABG:** Hypoxemia and hypercapnia (respiratory failure type 2)
- **X-ray for emphysema:** hyperinflation, diaphragm flattened

- **Blood:**
- Low a1 antitrypsin (emphysema)
- Polycythemia

- **Staging system:**
- GOLD (FEV1)
- BODE index
  (mortality & prognostic)
  Body mass index (BMI)
  Airflow obstruction (FEV1)
  Dyspnoea (MRCC)
  Exercise capacity (6 min walk distance)

- **Complications:**
- Pneumonia, pulmonary hypertension, cor pulmonale (leg swelling), pneumothorax, respiratory failure

- **Treatments:**
- Quit smoking
- Oxygen therapy: arterial Po2 <55 mm Hg or O2 saturation <88%
- Pulmonary rehabilitation
- Inhaled ipratropium (anticholinergic)
- Inhaled β2-agonists
- SABA

# Respiratory Examination

- **Surgery:**
  - Bullectomy for subpleural belb
  - lung transplant

**\* Long Term Oxygen Therapy (LTOT):**

-oxygen saturation is ≤88% or PaO <7.3 kPa at rest

-For 16 hr daily.

**Acute exacerbation of COPD:**

  a. Haemophilus influenzae ,Streptococcus pneumoniae or viral
  b. Managed by :
     -Oxygen, IV antibiotic ,Nebulized SABA and SAMA (terbutaline, ipratropium) ,PO steroid or IV hydrocortisone

*If above measure fail (PaCO2 increasing and PH decreasing ) do NIV (BiPap) , finally if NIV fail do endotracheal intubation .

## ❖ PNEUMOTHORAX

- **Types:**
A. **Spotuoues**:
1. **primary:** without any causes (tall thin young health patients ,smoking)
2. **Secondary:** respiratory pathology (copd)
B. **Tension**

- **Clinical features:**
- Unilateral chest pain
- Dyspnea at rest
- Hyperresonant
- Decreased breath sound
- Unstable (low BP ,tracheal deviation ,high JVP )

- **Investigations:**
- X-ray: visible visceral pleural line

# Respiratory Examination

❖ **Pulmonary fibrosis:**

- **Upper lobes (CHART_SS)**
  - coal
  - histiocytosis
  - ankylosing spondylitis
  - allergic bronchopulmonary aspergillosis
  - radiation
  - Tuberculosis
  - silicosis
  - sarcoidosis
- **Lower lobes (A RISO )**
  - Asbestosis
  - RA
  - IPF
  - Scleroderma
  - other ( methotrexate, amiodarone)

❖ **Idiopathic pulmonary fibrosis:**

- **Clinical features:**
  - progressive dyspnea
  - non-productive cough
- **Findings:**
  - bibasilar crackles ( end-inspiratory crackles)
  - cor pulmonale
  - clubbing
  - X-ray: ground-glass, honeycomb, reticular opacities
  - CT: fibrosis
  - Surgical lung biopsy
- **Treatment:**
  - Pirfenidone
  - Nintedanib
  - Steroid

❖ **Pleural effusion:**

- Reduced chest expansion on affected side
- Tracheal deviation(away)
- Stony dull
- Decreased vocal resonance
- Low or absent breath sounds

**CXR**: Blunting costophrenic angle

### Respiratory Examination

**Pleural** tap(diagnostic)

Complication Pleural tap or thoracentesis :

- Pneumothorax

-haemothorax

-pulmonary oedema

* Meigs syndrome :

right pleural effusion ascite & ovarian malignancy.


- **Exudative is determined by Light's criteria:**
- Pleural fluid protein / Serum protein >0.5
- Pleural fluid LDH / Serum LDH >0.6
- Pleural fluid LDH > 2/3 of Serum LDH Upper Limit of Normal

| Transudative | Exudative |
|---|---|
| • HF <br> • Hypoalbuminemia(cirrhosis , nephrotic syndrome) | • Infection(pneumonia) <br> • Malignancy <br> • RA <br> • Pancreatitis |


"bronchogenic carcinoma"

-Lung :Cough haemoptysis, &SOB

-generalized weight loss,anorexia

-Local pressure effects: recurrent laryngeal palsy, superior vena cava obstruction, Horner syndrome

- Endocrine (SIADH), hypercalcaemia(Pthrp), Cushing syndrome(Acth)

-Neurological: Eaton–Lambert syndrome

-Clubbing

# Respiratory Examination

**Cystic fibrosis**

**Clinical features:**
- Autosomal recessive
- Mutation in gene that code CFTR protein
- Sweat chloride test >60 mEq/L

- **Complication:**
1. Nasal polyp, sinusitis, bronchiectasis
2. Chronic pancreatitis, DM,
3. ADEK (vitamin deficiency) osteoporosis
4. meconium ileus, small intestinal stenosis or obstruction ileocecal valve
5. Bile duct obstruction
6. Infertility (male) due absence of vas deferens

- **5 Classes of CFTR mutation:**

| | | |
|---|---|---|
| 1 | - | Defect in protein production (no protein is made) |
| 2(F508) | - | Defective protein processing (trafficking) protein cannot make it to the membrane |
| 3(G551D) | - | Defective channel regulation (protein on membrane but not working at all) |
| 4 | - | Defective channel conductance (protein at membrane but not doing enough) (quality) |
| 5 | - | Decreased active CFTR (protein at membrane and working good but the number is low ) (quantity ) |

- **FEV1 indicates (severity)**
- Infection: by
  - S. aureus
  - Pseudomonas aeruginosa
  - Burkholderia

# Respiratory Examination

- Aspergillus

- **Treatment:**
- Inhaled bronchodilators and glucocorticoids for airway obstruction
- Ivacaftor (G551D)
- Chronic Pseudomonas Infection use nebulized (aztreonam, tobramycin)
- **Viscous is decreased by:**
- inhaled rhDNase, inhaled hypertonic (7%) saline
- Pancreatic enzyme, PPI
- ADEK vitamin
- chest physiotherapy

### ❖ Bronchiectasis:

- **Due**
- CF, recurrent infection, immunodeficiency

- **Clinical features:**
- Chronic productive cough, hemoptysis
- Crackles or rhonchi or wheezing on auscultation
- Clubbing
- CXR=Tram-track lines

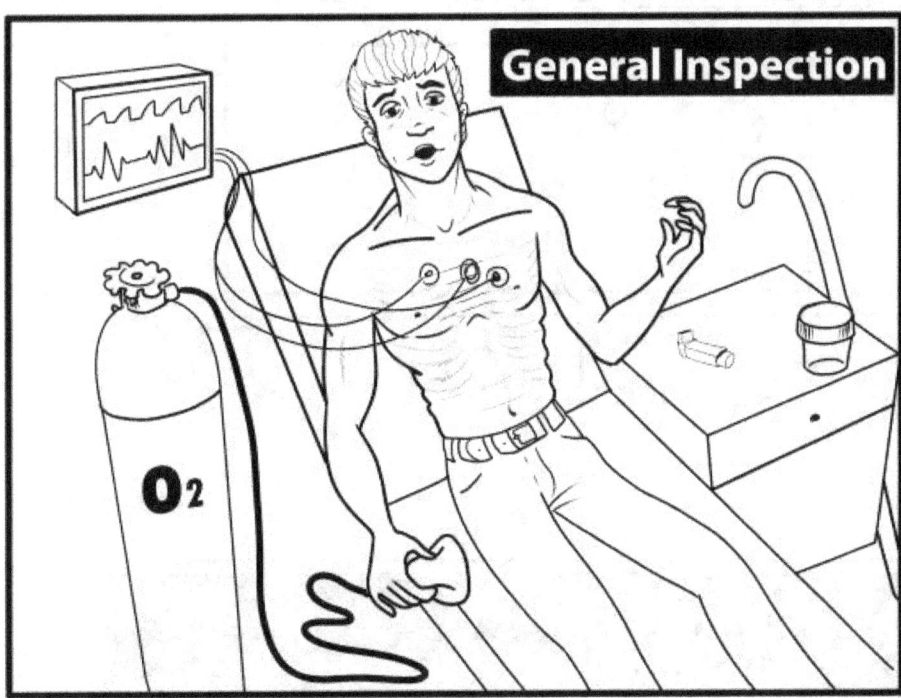

# Respiratory Examination

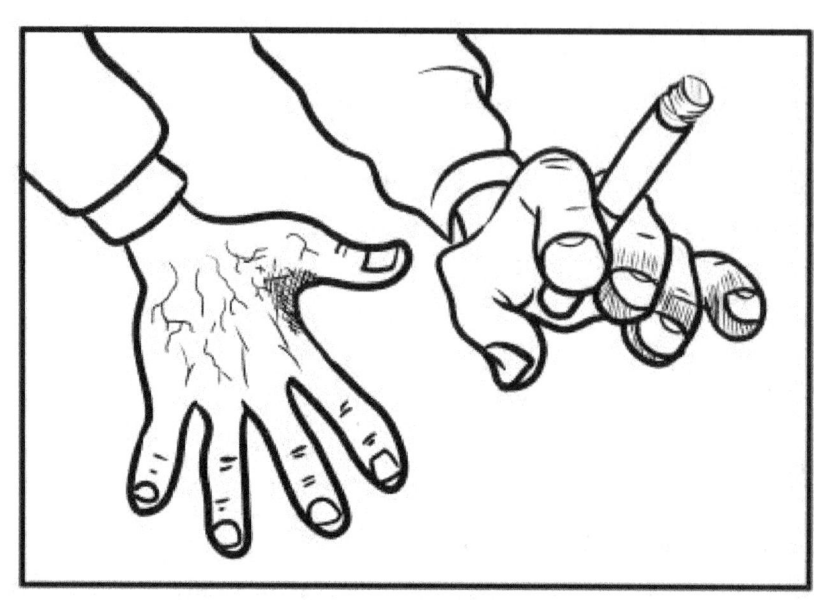

**Clubbing - Tar Stain - Peripheral Cyanosis - 1st Web Space Atrophy**

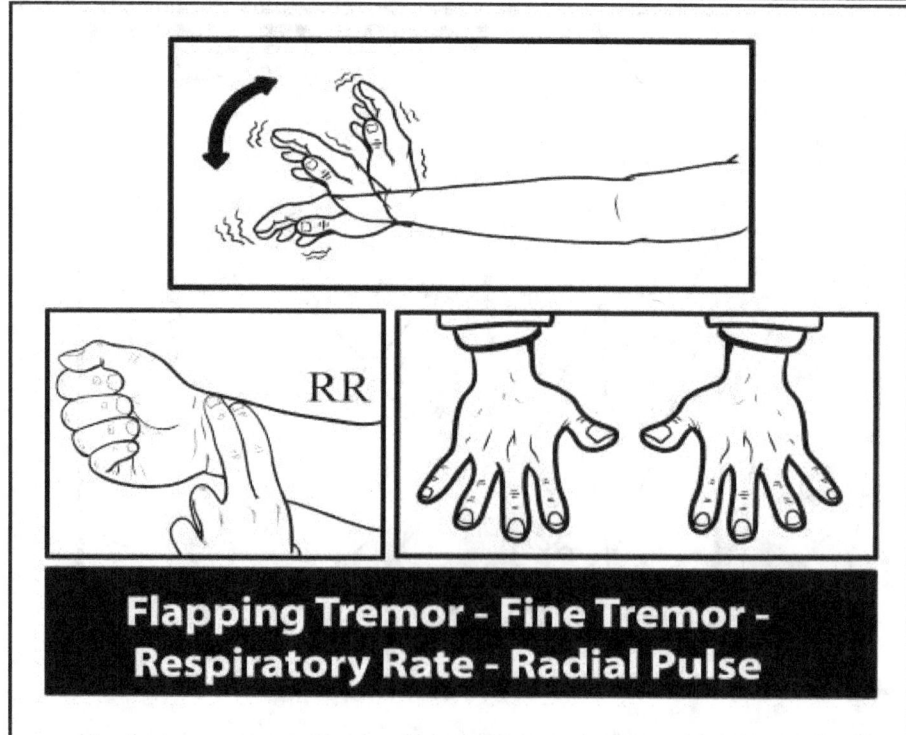

**Flapping Tremor - Fine Tremor - Respiratory Rate - Radial Pulse**

# Respiratory Examination

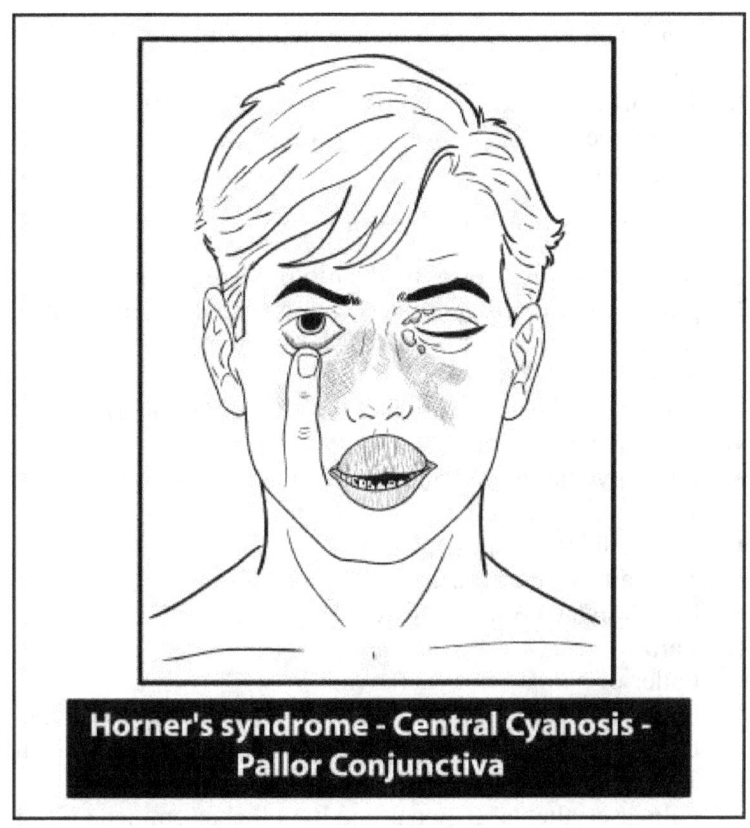

Horner's syndrome - Central Cyanosis - Pallor Conjunctiva

# GIT Examination

| | |
|---|---|
| **General** | 1. Wash hands, introduce yourself, name and age, explain your roles and gain permission<br>2. Top off till pubic symphysis is enough or ideally nipples to knees<br>3. 45 degrees for inspection and supine with one pillow behind head for palpation |
| **Inspection** | 1. **Around the bed:** drip, medications, nasogastric tube.<br>2. **patient:** confused or coma (hepatic encephalopathy), distress or cachexia (tumor, cirrhosis), BMI and jaundice<br>3. **Nails:**<br>• Clubbing (cirrhosis, Coeliac, IBD, GI lymphoma)<br>• Koilonychias (anemia)<br>• Leukonychia (hypoalbuminemia in nephrotic syndrome, celiac, kwashiorkor, CLD)<br>• Terry's lines (cirrhosis, DM)<br>• Tar stains (crohn, pancreatic tumor, PUD)<br>• Blue lunulae (Wilson's disease)<br>4. **Palm:**<br>• Pallor of palmar creases (anemia)<br>• Dupuytren's contracture (alcoholic liver disease, DM, familial) also feel palm for thickening of palmar fascia at fourth and fifth fingers<br>• Tendon xanthoma (hyperlipidemia, PBC)<br>• Palmar erythema in thenar and hypothenar eminences (CLD, pregnancy, hyperthyroidism, RA)<br>• Flapping tremor(Asterixis):<br>   - stretch out your hands<br>   - dorsiflexed your wrist<br>   - separate your fingers for 15 seconds<br>   - bilateral flap (hepatic encephalopathy)<br>5. **Arm:**<br>• Ecchymosis, petechiae (cirrhosis)<br>• Tattoo or needle marks (HBV, HCV)<br>• Spider naevi in distribution of SVC like arms, upper trunk, face more or equal than 5 is abnormally (high estrogen in pregnancy and CLD)<br>• Dermatitis herpetiformis extensor surface of arms and legs (celiac disease)<br>• Scratch marks (Cholestatic pruritus)<br>• Acanthosis Nigerians (GIT cancer)<br><br>6. **Eyes:**<br>• Scleral icterus(Jaundice)<br>• Conjunctival pallor(anemia) |

# GIT Examination

|  |  |
|---|---|
|  | - Kayser–Fleischer rings (Wilson disease)<br>- Episcleritis, conjunctivitis, uveitis(IBD)<br>- Xanthelasma, corneal arcus (hyperlipidemia)<br><br>**7. Mouth:**<br>- Angular cheilitis (iron deficiency)<br>- Lips pigmentation: Peutz-Jeghers disease (polyps in colon) +Addison disease<br>- Telangiectasia in lip (Rendu-Osler-Weber disease +++ with AV malformations causing GIT bleeding)<br>- Fetor hepaticus<br>- Aphthous ulcers (celiac, IBD)<br>- Oral candidiasis (steroid +immunocompromised)<br>- Glossitis (folate, vitamin B12 deficiency)<br>- Bilateral parotid enlargement (alcohol abuse or bulimia)<br><br>**8. Head and neck lymph nodes:**<br>- Left supraclavicular lymph enlargement (Virchow's node: gastric tumor)<br>- Generalized lymphadenopathy with hepatosplenomegaly (lymphoma)<br><br>**9. Abdomen:**<br>- Hernia: ask the patient to Cough<br>- Diastasis recti (Raise your head)<br>- (SSS)Scars stoma +Striate (white stretch marks, pink Cushing disease)<br>- Dilated veins:(IVC obstruction lateral vein, hepatic cirrhosis portal HTN, caput medusae)<br>- Grey tuner, Cullen sign(pancreatitis)<br>- Sister Mary Joseph nodule (GIT tumor)<br>- Gynecomastia + testicular atrophy + loss of axillary and suprapubic hair (high estrogen due cirrhosis)<br>- Distension (fat, fluid, foetus, facease, flatus)<br>- Abdominal wall is not moving with respiration (peritonitis) |
| **Palpation** | **1. Abdomen**<br>- Ask for pain (start away from pain)<br>- Rest your hand and only flex your MCP<br>- Light (tenderness)and deep palpation(masses) for 9 regions<br>- Watch patient face for Tenderness: generalized with rebound tenderness (peritonitis), epigastric (PUD), RHR(cholecystitis), RIR (appendicitis, crohn), LIR(diverticulitis) |

# GIT Examination

- Rigidity (generalized peritonitis)
- Masses: epigastric (pancreatic stomach tumors + AAA) + RIR (crohn, appendicitis abscess, proximal colon tumor, Ileocecal tuberculosis) LIR (diverticular diseases +sigmoid cancer)

2. **Liver**
   - Your fingers should be aligned in the same direction of right costal margin
   - Palpate during inspiration from RIR to right costal margin and along costal margin medially and laterally
   - If you feel liver edge:
   - enlargement by fingerbreadths from costal margin
   - **Normal:**
   - Riedel's lobe
   - COPF
   - **Abnormal:**
   - Tenderness (hepatitis, right heart failure)
   - Smooth (Hepatic steatosis)
   - Hard irregular nodular (metastasis, or cyst, HCC, Macronodular cirrhosis)
   - Bruits (HCC, alcoholic hepatitis, AV malformation)
   - Venous hum(cirrhosis)
   - Pulsatile (tricuspid reg)

3. **Spleen (9-11 rib)**
   - Your fingers should be aligned in the same direction of left costal margin.
   - Start from RIR to left costal margin during inspiration.
   - Other maneuver: two hand technique: one hand palpate while the other is pulling rib cage up or ask patient to lie on his right side

4. **Kidney:**
   - Bimanual palpation
   - Unilateral enlargement (cyst, hydronephrosis)
   - Bilateral (PKD)

5. **AAA:**
   - Place the tips of your hands between abdominal aorta above umbilicus
   - Transverse diameter less than 2–3cm (normal)
   - More than 3 cm aneurysm, more than 5 cm start treatment
   - Pulsatile and expandable(AAA)

# GIT Examination

| | |
|---|---|
| **Percussion** | 1. **liver:**<br>percuss from RIF in the mid clavicular line until resonance become dullness (lower border of the liver) then percuss right chest to find the upper border(dull)<br><br>2. **Spleen:** start from RIR till Left costal margin |
| **Ascites** | 1. **Shifting dullness:**<br>• Percuss from the umbilicus to the patient's left side until the resonance become dullness (leave your fingers here)<br>• Ask the patient to lay in right side<br>• Wait for 30 seconds<br>• Percuss again (previously dullness is now resonance)<br>• Ascites =positive<br><br>2. **Fluid thrill (large ascites):**<br>• Ask the patient to put the edge of his hand in midline<br>• Place your left hand palm in the left side of stomach the flick with your right hand against patient right abdomen<br>• Ascites= positive if thrill felt on the left hand |
| **Auscultation** | 1. Bowel sound in RIR for 2 min 5 to 34 per min<br>• no bowel sound=peritonitis, obstruction<br>2. Above umbilical for aortic bruit<br>3. 2-3 cm above and lateral to umbilicus for renal bruit(both renal arteries) |
| **Other** | • Legs:<br>- Pyoderma gangrenosum + erythema nodosum (IBD)<br>- Ankle oedema(hypoalbuminemia)<br>• Migratory thrombophlebitis (pancreatic tumor)<br>• Murphy sign(cholecystitis)<br>• Rovsing, psoas and obturator signs(Appendicitis)<br>• Courvoisier's law (pancreatic tumor) |
| **The end** | ➢ **External genitalia and groin:**<br>• Femoral hernia<br>• Testicular atrophy(cirrhosis)<br>• DRE (Bulmer's shelf (gastric met)<br>• Ovary (krukenberg tumor) |

# GIT Examination

❖ **Extraintestinal manifestations of IBD:**
- **Skin:** pyoderma gangrenosum, erythema nodosum
- **Joint:** peripheral arthritis, ankylosing spondylitis
- **Eye:** anterior uveitis, iritis, Episcleritis

❖ **Comparison of Crohn disease versus Ulcerative Colitis**

|  | **Crohn disease** | **Ulcerative Colitis** |
|---|---|---|
| **Site of Origin** | Terminal ileum | Rectum |
| **Pattern of Progression** | "skip" lesions/irregular | Proximally contiguous |
| **Thickness of Inflammation** | Transmural | Submucosa or mucosa |
| **Symptoms** | Crampy abdominal pain | Bloody diarrhea |
| **Complications** | Fistulas, abscess, obstructions | Hemorrhage, toxic megacolon |
| **Radiographic Findings** | String sign on barium X-ray | Lead pipe colon on barium X-ray |
| **Biopsy** | Granulomas | Crypt Abscess |

➢ **Treatment of IBD:**
- 5-ASA
- Anti TNF: infliximab or adalimumab
- Immunosuppressive drugs: azathioprine
- Oral or topical prednisone (acute attack)
- Antibiotic: Metronidazole

- Check thiopurine methyltransferase level before starting azathioprine or 6-MP, drugs toxicity is high if its low

➢ **Surgeries:**
- Total proctocolectomy with ileoanal anastomosis for UC
- Terminal ileum resection for Crohn's disease

➢ **Indications for surgery:**
- Abscess, fistula, stricture, fulminant colitis, toxic Megacolon, unresponsive to medication.
- Dysphagia : difficulty in swallowing
- Odynophagia: pain in swallowing
- Causes : bisphosphate , thrush (HIV), HSV, CMV

# GIT Examination

- **Dysphagia :**
  1. **Oropharyngeal**:(difficulty in initiating the swallowing )
     - Present as coughing, choking , regurgitating the food nasally.
     - For example: stroke, parkision, MG

  2. **Esophageal**:
     - **Solid** :
       a. Progressive : esophageal cancer , stricture from PUD
       b. Episodic : Plummer Vinson syndrome , rings

     - **Solid and liquid :**
       a. Achalasia:
       - "bird's beak" in barium swallow

  3. **Sclerosis**
     - Other esophageal spasm ,eosinophilic esophagitis , Left atrial dilation

❖ **hepatomegaly:**

| Infection | Inflammation | Metabolic |
|---|---|---|
| **Bacterial:**<br>- TB<br>**Viral:**<br>- EBV<br>- CMV<br>**Protozoal:**<br>- Malaria<br>- Histoplasmosis | • Hepatic steatosis<br>• Hepatitis<br>• PBC | • Wilson's disease<br>• Haemochromatosis amyloid |

| Malignant | Congestive |
|---|---|
| • HCC<br>• adenoma (OCP, steroid)<br>• METS<br>• Lymphoma<br>• Leukemia | • RHF<br>• Tricuspid regurgitation<br>• Budd-Chiari syndrome |

❖ **Splenomegaly:**

| Systemic | Liver | Haematological | Infective |
|---|---|---|---|
| | | | |

## GIT Examination

| | | | |
|---|---|---|---|
| • Amyloidosis<br>• Sarcoidosis<br>• Rheumatoid arthritis (felty syndrome) | • Portal hypertension (Cirrhosis) | • Haemolytic anemia<br>• Myeloproliferative disorders (myelofibrosis)<br>• Sickle cell disease / thalassemia<br>• Leukaemia<br>• Lymphoma | • EBV, CMV<br>• Malaria<br>• Brucella - leishmaniasis (Kala-Azar)<br>• schistosomiasis |

➢ **GIT bleeding:**

| Upper GI Bleeding | Lower GI Bleeding |
|---|---|
| • PUD<br>• Gastritis<br>• Esophageal cancer<br>• Mallory Weiss tear<br>• Varices | • Angiodysplasia (++ aortic stenosis)<br>• Diverticulosis<br>• Polyps<br>• IBD<br>• Cancer<br>• Hemorrhoids |

**Obstruction:**

| SBO | LBO |
|---|---|
| • **Due**: hernia, adhesion, stoma, volvulus<br>• **X-ray**: >3cm(dilation)<br>• **Central location** (ladders like dilation)<br>• valvulae conniventes | • **Due**: colon tumor, stricture, IBD, Sigmoid volvulus<br>• **X-ray:** >6 cm(dilation)<br>• **Peripheral location** (picture frame)<br>• Haustration |

# GIT Examination

➢ **Cirrhosis:**
- **Clinical picture :**
- Jaundice, fatigue
- Hyperestrogenism:
- Gynecomastia, loss of body hair , palmar erythema , spider naevi ,testicular atrophy,ED ,infertility
- Hepatorenal syndrome(increased Cr)
- Hepatopulmonary syndrome (SOB)
- Hepatic Osteodystrophy (osteoporosis)
- Hepatic encephalopathy (Asterixis )
- Portal hypertension:
- Lab:Low albumin , high bilirubin , high INR , low platelet (petechiae )

Grading system :Childs–Pugh classification(prognostic)
INR , bilirubin, albumin ,encephalopathy, ascites

a. **Ascite** (also due hypoalbuminemia ): paracentesis
1. Ascetic Fluid Protein:<2.5 g/dL
2. SAAG >1.1
3. SBP:PMN>250/µL c
b. **Splenomegaly**
c. **Hypersplenism** (low Plt. )
d. **Caput medusae**
e. **Varicella hemorrhage**
f. **hemorrhoids**

| Ascites | Causes | Treatment |
|---|---|---|
| • T=Transudate<br>• E=Exudate | • **Liver:**<br>- CLD(cirrhosis)(T)<br>- Budd-Chiari syndrome(T)<br>- IVC obstruction(T)<br>• **Heart:**<br>- RHF(T)<br>- Abdominal tumor(E)<br>- Nephrotic syndrome(E)<br>- TB(E)<br>- Meigs syndrome | • Low salt diet<br>• WT loss<br>• Diuretic<br>• Therapeutic paracentesis<br>• TIPS<br>• Le Veen shunt |

-**WILSON'S DISEASE**(copper overload)

- tremor and hepatomegaly,jaundice

## GIT Examination

-Kayser–Fleischer ring

-**HAEMOCHROMATOSIS**(iron overload):

-Pronze(tan)skin ,DM2 , restrictive cardiomyopathy , pseudogout, osteoporosis , hypopituitarism (testicular atrophy )

- Transferrin saturation &  Serum ferritin are high

**PRIMARY BILIARY CIRRHOSIS:**

-Female fatigue and pruritus

-Xanthelasma

-Jaundice

-Scratch marks

*High ALP , IgM , AMA

*Associated with autoimmune disease :Sicca syndrome , RA, hashimoto's hypothyroidism

*Celiac diseases*:

Small intestine biopsy (villous atrophy/blunted )

IgA Anti-tissue Transglutaminase Antibodies

Anti-endomysial antibody (EMA)

Complication:

      a. Anemia (normocytic , macrocytic,or both )
      b. Dermatitis herpetiformis :<u>itchy vesicles *extensor*</u> surface
      c. **MALT** lymphoma
      d. Vitamin deficiency  ADEK
      e. Functional asplenia

**Gynecomastia**

-Testicular failure : Klinefelter's, viral orchitis

-Estrogen effect: CLD, thyrotox

## GIT Examination

-Drug-induced :spironolactone

-Marijuana

**Jaundice**

| Pre-hepatic | Hepatic | Post-hepatic |
|---|---|---|
| -Haemolytic anaemia<br><br>-Gilbert's syndrome - Criggler-Najjar syndrome | -Alcoholic liver disease<br><br>-Viral hepatitis<br><br>-NAFLD<br><br>-inflammatory ( Hereditary haemochromatosis,wilson disease)<br><br>-Autoimmune hepatitis<br><br>Primary biliary cirrhosis<br><br>-Hepatocellular carcinoma | -Choledocholithiasis<br><br>-pancreatic cancer<br><br>-biliary duct strictures<br><br>-cholangiocarcinoma |

# GIT Examination

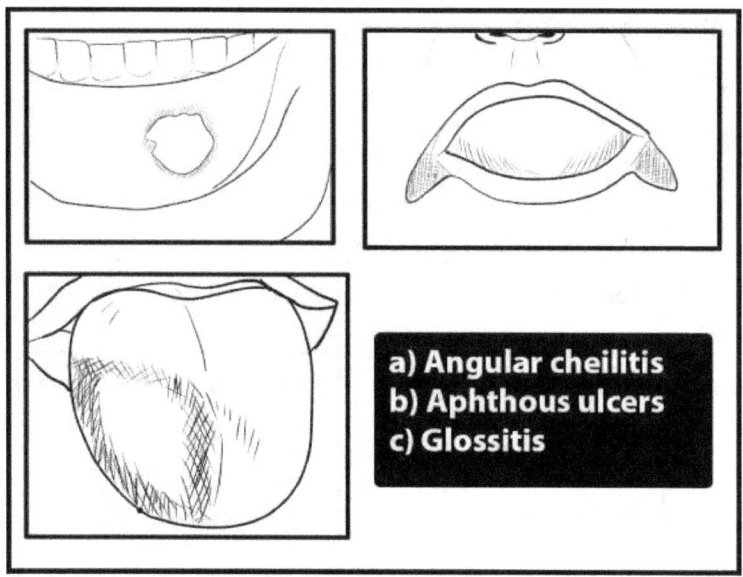

a) Angular cheilitis
b) Aphthous ulcers
c) Glossitis

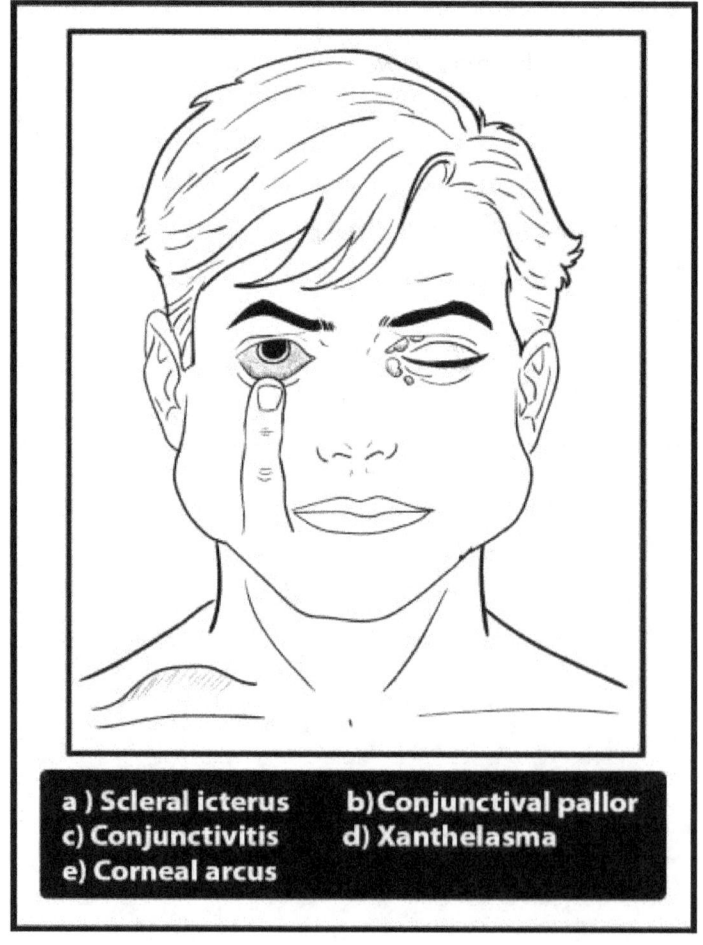

a) Scleral icterus    b) Conjunctival pallor
c) Conjunctivitis     d) Xanthelasma
e) Corneal arcus

# GIT Examination

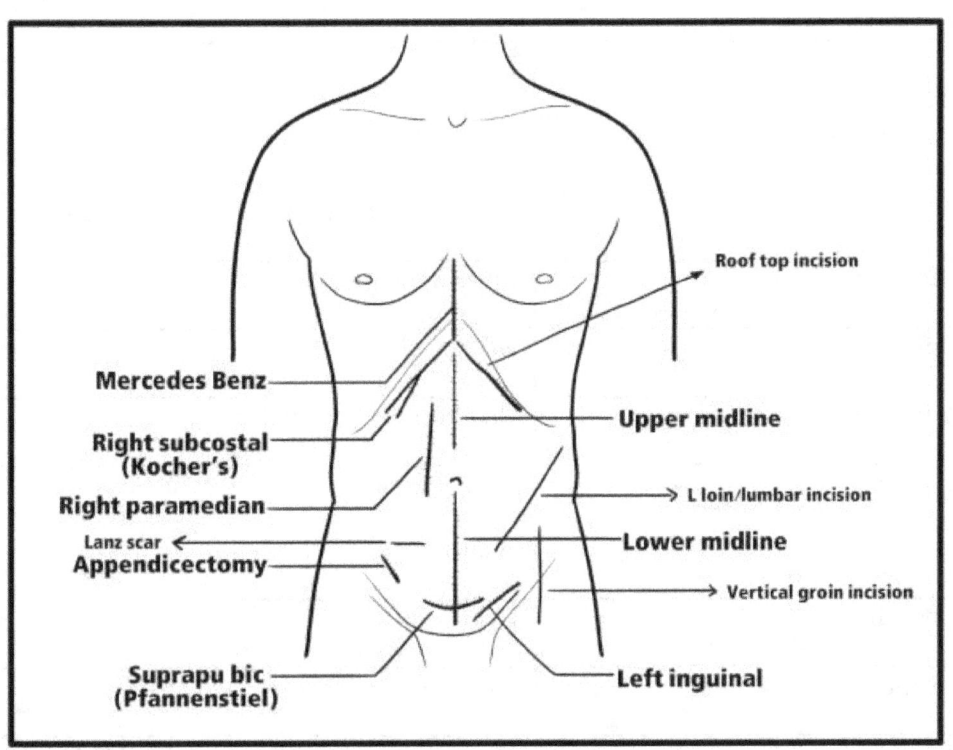

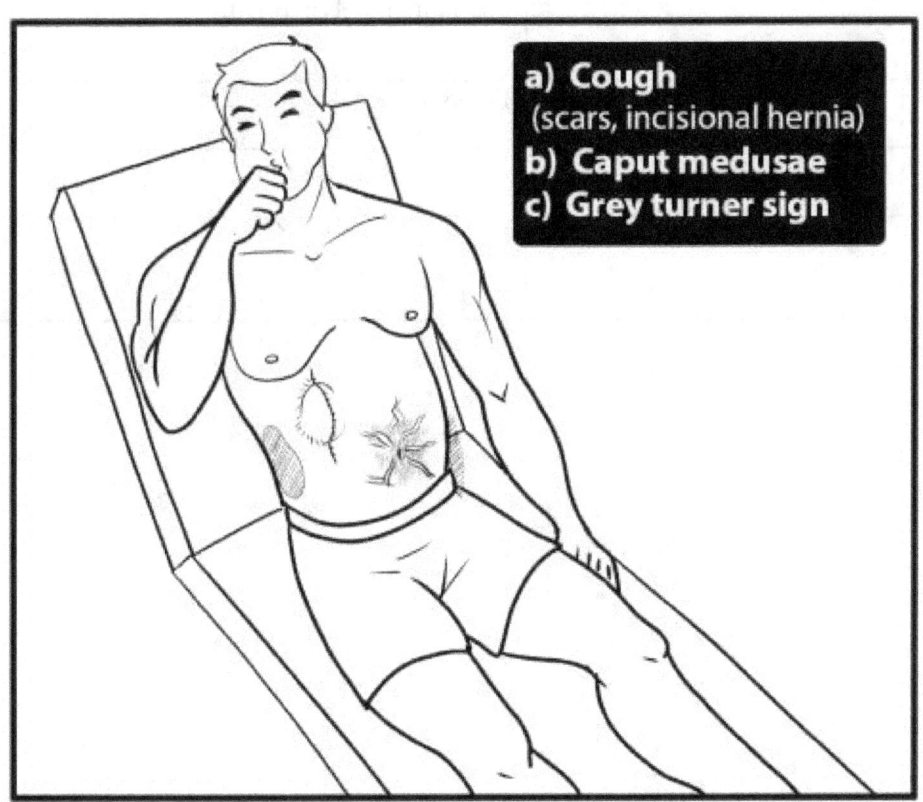

## GIT Examination

| **Lanz**<br>**Point scar**<br>**Gridiron(appendectomy) incisions** | **Appendectomy** |
|---|---|
| Kochar(subcostal)incision | Cholecystectomy |
| Mercedes-Benz scars | Liver transplant |
| Renal transplant | Hockey stick |
| Lateral lumbar scar | Nephrectomy, renal surgery |
| Left Paramedian | Anterior rectal resection, colectomy laparotomy |
| Right Paramedian | Hemicolectomy |
| Transverse suprapubic | Hysterectomy |
| Midline | laparotomy (general surgery for AAA, abdominal, pelvic organ) |
| Vertical groin | Femoral vessels |
| Oblique groin | Inguinal canal (hernia) |
| Point scar | Laparoscopy |

# GIT Examination

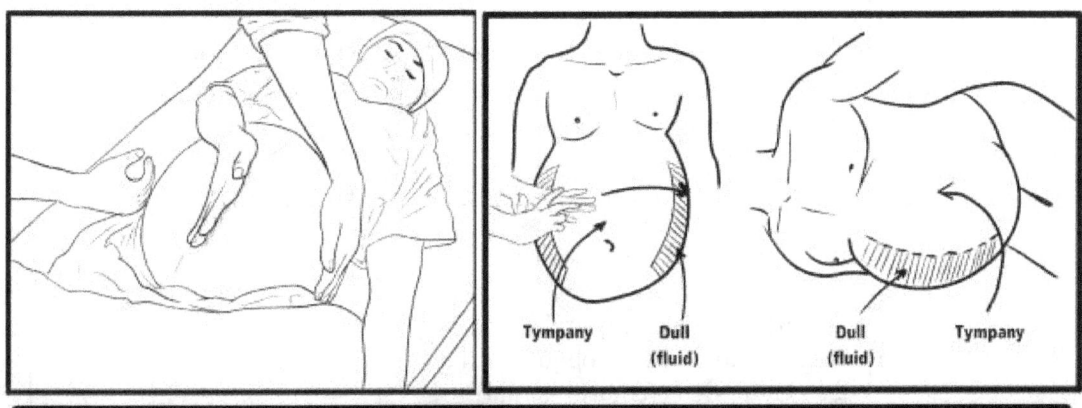

- Fluid thrill          - Shifting dullness

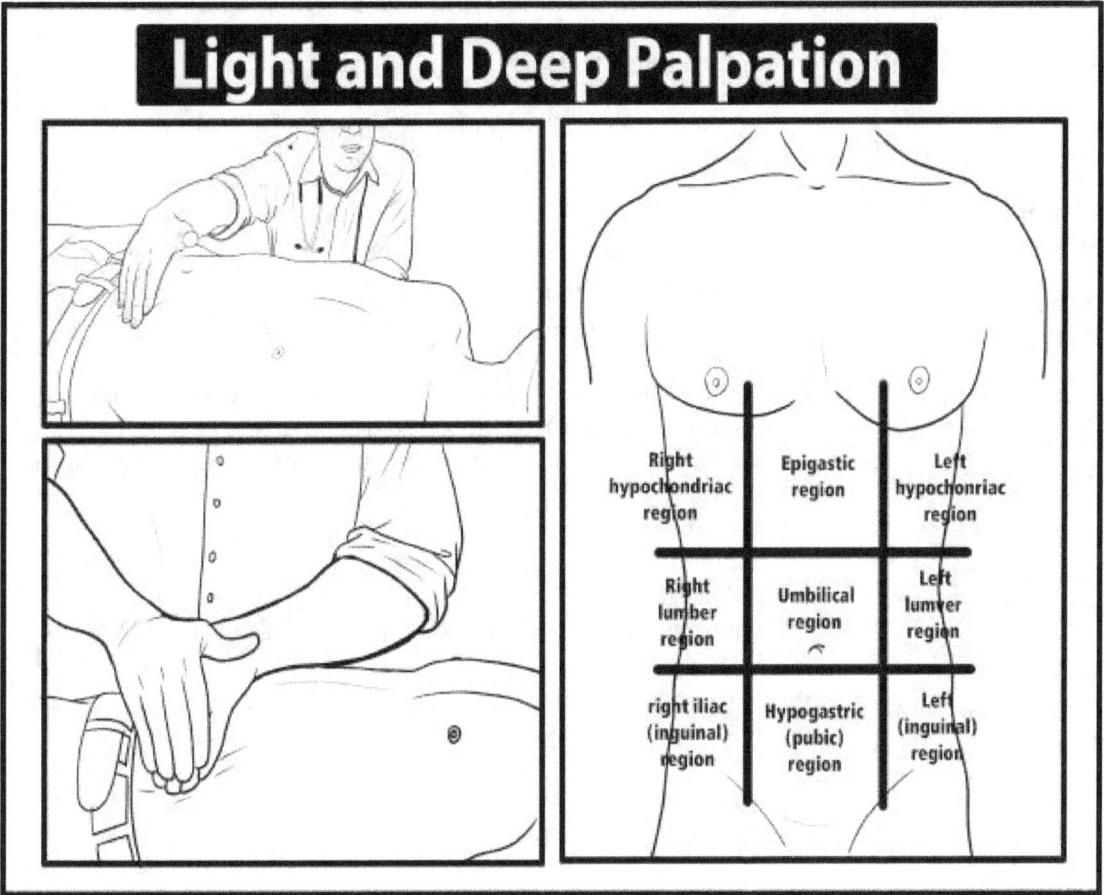

## Hernia & Stoma Examination

| | |
|---|---|
| **General** | 1. A continuous of the GIT examination but patient<br>2. Ask the Pt to cough if the lump is not obvious<br>3. Ask Pt to stand up if its still not obvious |
| **Inspection** | 1. Scars (incisional hernia)<br>2. Obvious lumb<br>3. Scrotal swelling (indirect hernia)<br>4. Ask to Cough (cough impulse)<br>5. Gaur sign (femoral hernia)<br>6. Scrotal swelling<br>7. Skin over hernia (redness) strangulated |
| **Palpate**<br><br>**Differential diagnosis**<br><br>• **Above inguinal ligament:**<br>- Inguinal lymphadenopathy<br>- ectopic testis<br>- Malgaigne's bulgings<br>• **below:**<br>- Saphena varix<br>- Femoral Aneurysm<br>• **both**:<br>- Muscle abscess<br>- Lipoma<br>- Cyst | 1. **Cough impulse test:**<br>• put your two fingers above<br>• ask patient to cough feel for impulse<br>• negative for femoral and strangulated hernia<br><br>2. **palpate swelling**<br>- Describe lumb in term of location<br>a) Inguinal hernias superomedial pubic tubercle (above inguinal ligament)<br>b) Femoral hernias infralateral inguinal pubic tubercle (below inguinal ligament) Tenderness(strangulated), temperature (back of your hand) as in breast lump description (4S,4Tb, FCM)<br>3. **Reducibility**:<br>• supine if not reduced, either you or the patient himself reduce it<br>• with two fingers, put stress in midpoint of inguinal ligament<br>• ask patient to cough<br>• Reappearance of swelling (direct hernia), not (indirect hernia)<br>4. **Palpate scrotal for any swelling**<br>- extension of indirect hernia |

## Hernia & Stoma Examination

| | |
|---|---|
| Other | 1. **Auscultate(content)**<br>• Bowel sounds(gut)<br>• No sound (omentum or bowel obstruction)<br><br>2. **percussion**<br>• Resonant(gut)<br>• dull(omentum)<br>3. **Zieman's test:**<br>• using your three middle fingers:<br>  - Middle finger above external Inguinal Ring (direct hernia)<br>  - Index finger above internal Inguinal Ring (indirect hernia)<br>  - Ring finger above femoral canal (femoral hernia)<br>• then ask patient to cough<br>• the finger that elevates indicates the type of hernia |
| The End | - Offer full GIT examination |

❖ **Hernia:** protrusion of an organ through a defect in the wall of the cavity that contained this organ.

❖ **Causes:**

1. Increased intra-abdominal pressure(COPD,Chronic cough) ,constipation lifting, pregnancy,organomegaly,Obesity, ascites
2. Scars
3. Congenital (patent processes vaginalis)

❖ **Inguinal canal:**

- **Contents**: spermatic cord male), round ligament (female)
- **Internal ring** (mid inguinal ligament), external ring (superolateral to pubic tubercle)
- **Walls:**
1. **Anterior**: Aponeurosis of external oblique Aponeurosis of internal oblique(medially)
2. **Posterior**: Transversalis fascia conjoint Tendon(medially)
3. **Floor**: inguinal Ligament, lacunar Ligament(medially)
4. **Roof**: internal oblique Muscle transverse abdominus Muscle

# Hernia & Stoma Examination

❖ **Terms:**

- Irreducible hernia: cannot be returned to the abdominal cavity
- Obstructed hernia: irreducible hernia but blood supply fine
- Strangulated hernia: blood supply to the hernia blocked
- Complications of strangulated hernia: sepsis, bowel infarction, peritonitis, stricture
- Richter's hernia: part of bowel wall is strangulated but lumen is patent(obstructed but not strangulated hernia)
- mid-inguinal point : ½ between ASIS and symphysis puibis (femoral artery)
- midpoint of inguinal ligament :1/2 between ASIS AND PUIBIC TUBERCLE

| Indirect inguinal | Direct inguinal | Femoral hernia |
|---|---|---|
| • Bulges through the internal ring<br>• Travel into inguinal canal into external ring and enter the scrotum<br>• Neck is lateral to inferior epigastric artery,<br>• Younger men | • Muscle weakness in the posterior wall of the inguinal canal<br>• Neck is medial to inferior epigastric artery<br>• Through **Hesselbach's triangle**: borders:<br>- **medially**: rectus abdominis,<br>- **laterally**: inferior epigastric artery<br>- **Inferiorly**: inguinal ligament<br>• Older Male<br>• Bilateral<br>• Rarely strangulate and usually reducible by itself when Pt lying down | • Bulges through the femoral ring (opening of femoral canal)<br>• Femoral canal borders:<br>- **Medially:** lacunar ligament<br>- **lateral**: femoral vein<br>- **Anteriorly:** the inguinal ligament<br>- **Posteriorly:** Pectineal ligament<br>• **High risk of:** Strangulation and Irreducibility<br>• Female |

❖ **Management:**

- Trusses for patient unfit for surgery

-The aim is the strengthening of inguinal canal posterior wall

with synthetic mesh or without(bringing defect border together=posterior repair)

- o Open surgeries:
    - **Lichtenstein repair**: (mesh )

# Hernia & Stoma Examination

- **Shouldice repair:** (without mesh)
    - Laparoscopic surgeries (for bilateral or recurrent hernia)
        - Transabdominal preperitoneal repair (TAPP)(mesh)
        - Total extraperitoneal repair (TEP)(without mesh)
- **Complications:**
- Urinary retention, Pain (Ilioinguinal neuralgia, genitofemoral neuralgia)
- Haematoma, Infection
- Ischaemic orchitis, Scrotal swelling
- Recurrence

1. **Femoral hernia by three approaches:**
- **Lockwood**: below inguinal ligament
- **Lotheissen**: through inguinal canal
- **Mcevedy**: above inguinal canal

| Incisional hernia | Epigastric Hernia |
|---|---|
| <ul><li>Through scar</li><li>Risk factors:</li><li>a) midline scar</li><li>b) Dysfunctional wound healing (elderly, obesity, poor wound closure, steroid, DM)</li><li>c) Postoperative Haematoma, infection</li><li>Reducible specially in supine in position but swelling more prominent in standing)</li></ul> | <ul><li>Through linea alba</li><li>In midline between umbilicus and xiphisternum</li><li>Fat content</li></ul> |

| Paraumbilical Hernia | Umbilical hernia | Spigelian hernia |
|---|---|---|
| <ul><li>Through linea alba, just superior, inferior, medial, lateral to umbilicus</li><li>Umbilicus (crescent shape)</li><li>Strangulation (high)</li></ul> | <ul><li>Through umbilicus</li><li>Umbilicus (everted)</li><li>Congenital, ascites</li></ul> | <ul><li>Through arcuate line (lateral to rectus muscle)</li><li>Below umbilicus</li><li>Strangulation (high)</li></ul> |

- **Femoral canal :**
1. **Medial**: lacunar ligament
2. **Lateral**: femoral vein

3. **Anterior** :inguinal ligament
4. **Posterior** :pectineal ligament

❖ **Stoma**

## Hernia & Stoma Examination

| | |
|---|---|
| **General** | - A continuous of the GIT examination<br>- The same positioning and exposure<br>- Wear gloves, rule out any pain |
| **Inspection**<br>**LLSSCCC** | - Location (RIF, LIF, other)<br>- Lumen(opening numbers)<br>- Spouted or flushed to skin<br>- Skin around stoma (healthy or inflammation)<br>- Contents of stoma bag: watery (diarrhea, urine, hard stool)<br>- Complications<br>- Cough impulse test (parastomal hernia)<br>  Ask the Pt to cough |
| **Palpate and auscultate** | - Palpate for cough impulse using your hands around stoma<br>- Surround the stoma with your index fingers and thumbs<br>- Feel for tenderness around<br>- auscultation of bowel sound (obstruction) high-pitched tinkling sounds |
| **The End** | - Present your findings with what you think is likely the underlying pathology<br>- end colostomy: Ask if anus is closed or removed (Abdominoperineal resection) |

❖ **location for stoma:**

- **Through rectus muscle and easily accessible by patient**
- **Away from followings:**
- (USB)
- umbilicus
- scars
- skin creases
- bones (ribs, iliac crest)
- beltline

## Hernia & Stoma Examination

- **Complications:**
- **Outside the stoma**
  - Skin irritation (pyoderma gangrenosum)
  - Parastomal herniation
  - Small bowel obstruction
- **Stomal:**
  - Stenosis: managed by balloon dilation ,resection of the stenosed part.
  - Prolapse
  - Retraction: reoperation unless risk of peritonitis
  - Infection
  - Bleeding
  - necrosis(ischemia): color changes from red , moist into grey , pale , black
- **Other**
  - Electrolyte imbalances (dehydration high output)
  - Malabsorption
  - Short gut syndrome

|  | Purposes & Procedures | Features |
|---|---|---|
| **End colostomy** | • **Distal colon pathology:**<br>1. Obstruction (tumor, sigmoid volvulus)<br>2. Diverticulitis<br>3. Perforation<br>4. Ischemia<br>5. Fecal incontinence<br>6. Crohn's disease<br>• **Procedures**:<br>a) Sigmoid colon and upper rectum pathology:<br>- Hartmann's operation (emergency, reversible)<br>b) Low Rectum or anal cancer<br>- Abdominoperineal resection | 1. LIF<br>2. single lumen<br>3. Flush with skin<br>4. Content (bag): solid |
| **Loop colostomy** | • **Purposes**: same as end colostomy<br>• **temporary solutions** | • Same as end colostomy but two lumens, above umbilicus abdomen |
| **Double barreled colostomy** | • temporary | • Same as end colostomy but the two lumens separated (not joined) |
|  |  |  |

**Hernia & Stoma Examination**

| End ileostomy | • Proctocolectomy (ulcerative colitis ,FAP,tumor)<br>• Total colectomy | 1. RIF<br>2. Single lumen<br>3. Spouted<br>4. content: liquid |
|---|---|---|
| loop ileostomy | • Temporary( Acute Diverticulitis,Crohn's disease, protect newly made anastomosis) | • Same but two lumen |
| Urostomy | • Bladder disorder: (cystectomy, Neurogenic bladder),urinary incontinence | 1. One lumen<br>2. Spout(small)<br>3. Left or right |

❖ **Adenocarcinoma of colon:**
- **Location**
    - **Proximal** =bleeding ,anemia
    - **Distal**: obstruction ,perforation
    - **Rectal** : tenesmus ,decreased size of stool caliper

- **Tumor marker : CEA**
    - Colonoscopy (diagnostic)
    - Endoscopic USS/MRI for staging of rectal tumor

- **Classification by duke or TNM**
    - Stage I cancers penetrate into but not through the bowel wall
    - stage II cancers penetrate through the wall
    - stage III cancers involve regional lymph nodes
    - Stage IV metastases

1. **End colectomy :**
a. **Hartmann procedure :**
   - temporary solution
   - pathology in upper rectum and sigmoid so its removed
   - lower rectum and anal canal is still there
   - indication is in emergency (obstruction , diverticulitis ,perforation, sigmoid cancer )
   - can be reversed afterward (anus still there)
b. **AP resection :**
   - anus ,sigmoid , rectum removed
   - indication: rectal ca which is within 5 cm from the anal verge ,Crohn's proctitis with anal fistula ,recurrent/ residual anal SCC

## Hernia & Stoma Examination

- Permanent End Colostomy(anus is gone )
- anus is covered by Pedicled VRAM Flap – Pedicled Vertical Rectus Abdominis Myocutaneous Flap(look for the flap)

2. **End ileostomy :**
a. **Panproctocolectomy**
- from anus till cecum is removed
- Indication FAP ,UC , crohn ,HNPCC ,acromegaly
- Pt can pass stool again by anus : ileostomy can be reversed by J pouch

b. **Total Colectomy**
- large intestine remove except rectum and anal stump
- Emergency For UC (unresponsive for medication), Toxic Megacolon
- After surgery Pt ended up with end ileostomy and rectum and anal are still there
- Pt can pass stool again by anus :
- Topical steroid and 5-ASA for rectum then in few days do ileocecal anastomosis (connect small intestine to rectum)

3. **loop ileostomy**
- anterior resection
- only rectum+/-sigmoid is removed but anus is still there
- anastomosis is made between the remaining colon and anus but need time to heal so loop ileostomy is made temporary till anus is back to action

# Hernia & Stoma Examination

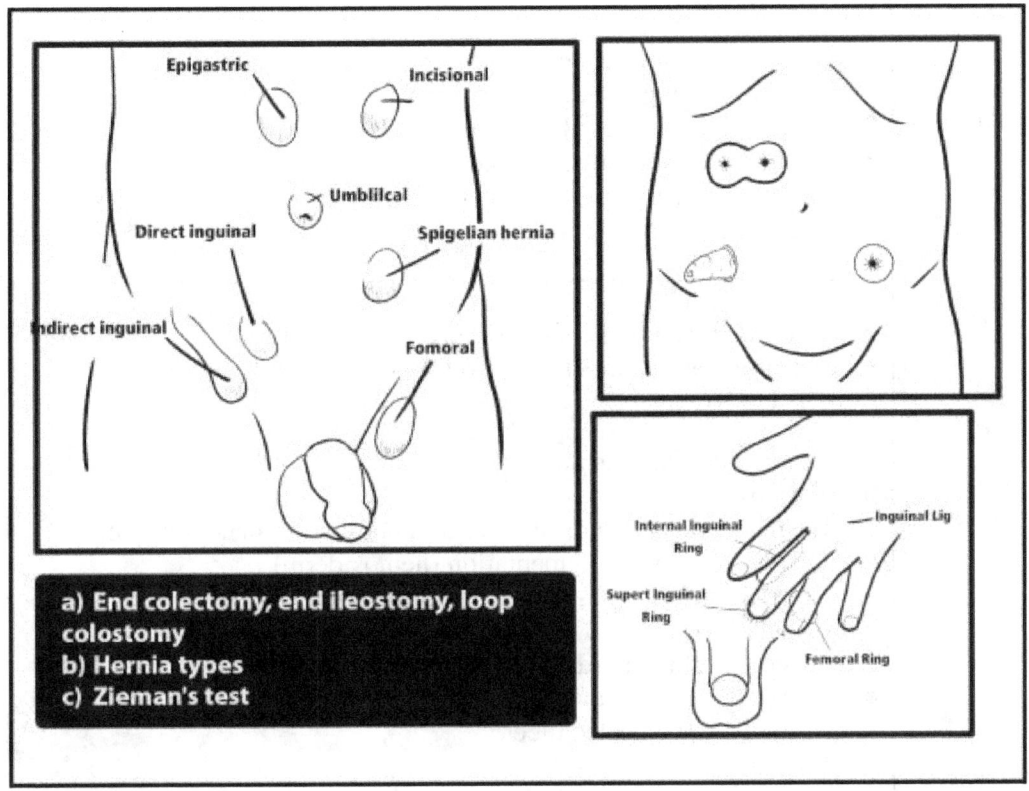
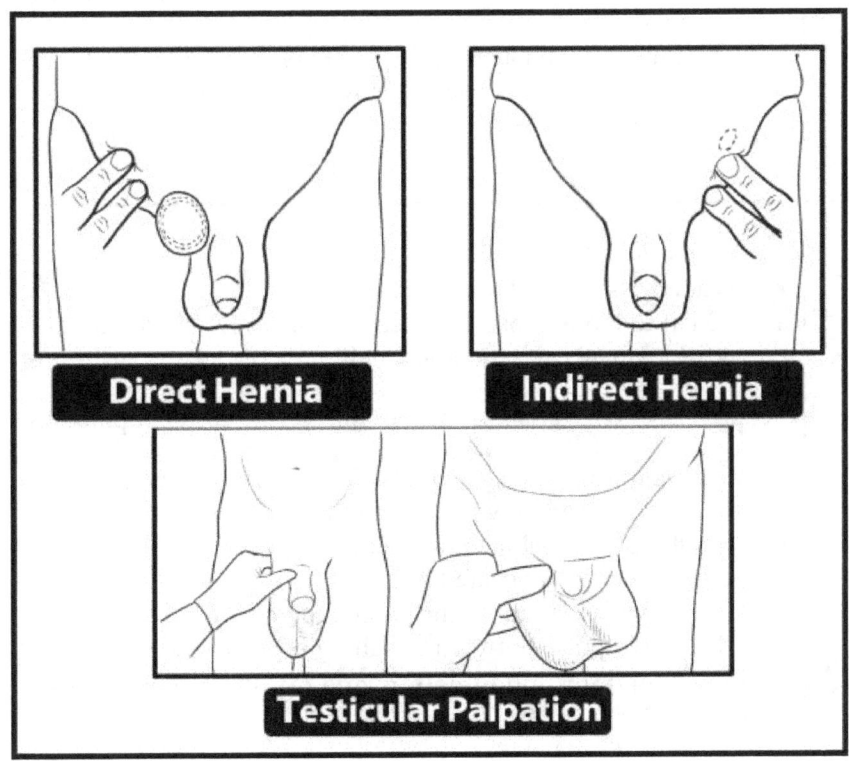

## Venous Vascular Examination

| | |
|---|---|
| **General** | 1. Wash hands, introduce yourself, get name and age, explain your roles and gain permission<br>2. standing, legs exposed (wearing shorts)<br>3. Around bed: walking aid, medicine<br>4. Patient: pain, Weight, pregnant, PE (SOB, pleurisy, haemoptysis, chest pain) |
| **Inspection** | • **Look between toes, back of foot**<br>• **Chronic venous insufficiency(CVI) :**<br>from bad to worse<br><br>a. Telangiectasia, reticular vein<br>b. Varicose veins<br>c. Edema (disappearance of veins and bony prominences in foot)<br>d. Eczema, brownish pigmentation (hemosiderin), Lipodermatosclerosis (inverted champagne bottle) atrophie blanche,<br>e. Ulcer (size, site, border, floor , exudate )<br>• Erythema: DVT, superficial thrombophlebitis<br>• Scars: surgery, healed ulcer<br>• DVT:<br>a. Phlegmasia cerulea dolens: bluish edematous painful leg with petechia<br>b. Phlegmasia alba dolens: pale pulseless cold leg<br>• Ankle flares: DVT, varicose vein<br>• Saphena varix at SFJ |
| **Palpation** | • Edema<br>• Tenderness<br>a. medial to femoral pulse tenderness due to DVT iliofemoral vein<br>Fingertips palpate calf tenderness calf vein(DVT)<br><br>Tender Cords over great saphenous superficial thrombophlebitis<br><br>• Temperature: both legs with back of hands (superficial thrombophlebitis, DVT, cellulitis)<br>• Cough test for SFJ incompetence:<br>- fingers over SFJ : located 2.5 cm below and lateral to the pubic tubercle(varics)<br>- Thrill or impulse felt with coughing is positive sign<br>* superficial thrombophlebitis due DVT, varicose veins |

## Venous Vascular Examination

| | |
|---|---|
| **Special Tests** | • **Venous tap or schwartz test:**<br>- percuss the distal part of LSV and feel the impulse on your left hand over the proximal part of LSV (patient standing)<br>- Impulse =positive for incompetence valves of LSV<br><br>• **Trendelenburg(Tourniquet) test:**<br>- PT supine 180 degrees<br>- Raise leg 90 degrees<br>- Empty superficial vein<br>- Apply tourniquet around SFJ<br>- Then stand up and notice for 30 sec<br><br>• **Findings:**<br>a. Superficial veins are still empty and when tourniquet is removed fill rapidly = SFJ incompetence<br>b. Superficial veins are filled despite tourniquet =perforator veins incompetence<br>• Perthes test: deep vein incompetence<br>- Apply tourniquet at SFJ and walk for few minuets<br>- Positive if any pain, superficial vein distention<br>• Homans sign(DVT)<br>• Auscultate varicose vein for bruit (AV fistula) |
| **The End** | • Doppler US(reflux)<br>• Examinations<br>a. Lower limb arterial examination<br>b. Abdominal examination (tumor) |

❖ **Lower limb venous system:**

1. **Superficial Veins:**
a. **greater saphenous vein:** above medial mallus to saphenofemoral junction
b. **lesser saphenous:** below lateral malleolus to popliteal fossa or above it
2. Deep veins (accompany arteries)
3. Perforating veins: connect both superficial and deep veins
4. Distal to proximal along the greater saphenous vein
a. Cockett (three prefoetrer at 3 different level above 5, 10, and 15 cm medial malleolus )
b. Boyd perforator: knee
c. Dodd perforator: distal thigh
d. Hunterian perforator: mid-thigh
e. Saphenofemoral junction

# Venous Vascular Examination

## ❖ CEAP Classification chronic venous disorders

|  | Chronic venous insufficiency (CVI) | DVT (common calf vein) |
|---|---|---|
| **Causes** | <ul><li>DVT</li><li>Varicose vein:</li></ul>a. Primary (idiopathic, familial):<br>b. Valvular defects<br>c. Secondary:<br>1. Pregnancy<br>2. AV fistula<br>3. Klippel-Trenaunay syndrome<br>4. Pelvic veins obstruction (abdominal or Pelvic tumor, LDP)<br>5. DVT causes incompetent vein valves (Post-Thrombotic Syndrome)<br>d. Congenital<br>- **Classifications:**<br>- CEAP system | <ul><li>Virchow triad (Hypercoagulability, Endothelial injury, stasis blood flow)</li><li>Tumor</li><li>Immobility (obesity, surgery, long-haul flight, fracture)</li><li>OCP, pregnancy</li></ul> |
| **Clinical Features** | <ul><li>Pain, edema, feeling of heavy leg worsens at night, improves by elevation</li><li>Telangiectasia, reticular vein</li><li>Brownish pigmentation (hemosiderin)</li><li>Lipodermatosclerosis (inverted champagne bottle) -stiffness (fibrosis</li><li>Eczema (scratches)</li><li>Atrophie blanche</li><li>Ulcer</li><li>Rule out DVT</li><li>Duplex US: venous reflux</li><li>And rule out any abdominal mass</li></ul> | <ul><li>Calf pain increases with walking and improves with rest</li><li>Swelling</li></ul>**Progression:**<br>- PE<br>- May-Thurner syndrome<br>- CVI<ul><li>WELL score</li><li>D-dimer</li><li>Duplex US</li><li>Contrast venography</li><li>MRI (venous veins)</li></ul> |
| **Treatment** | **Treatment according to etiology**<ul><li>Dressing and Unna boot for ulcer</li><li>Varicose vein:</li></ul>a. Compression stockings<br>b. Leg elevation<br>c. sclerotherapy injections or foams<br>d. < 3-4mm (telangiectasia +reticular vein)<br>e. EVLA, VNUS<br>f. Perforator incompetence: SEPS | <ul><li>LMWH + warfarin</li></ul> |

# Venous Vascular Examination

g. SFJ incompetence : Trendelenburg's operation and stripping(greater saphenous vein
- **complications**:
- Dysarthria ,pain :saphenous nerve GSV, sural nerve LSV
- Hematoma
- DVT

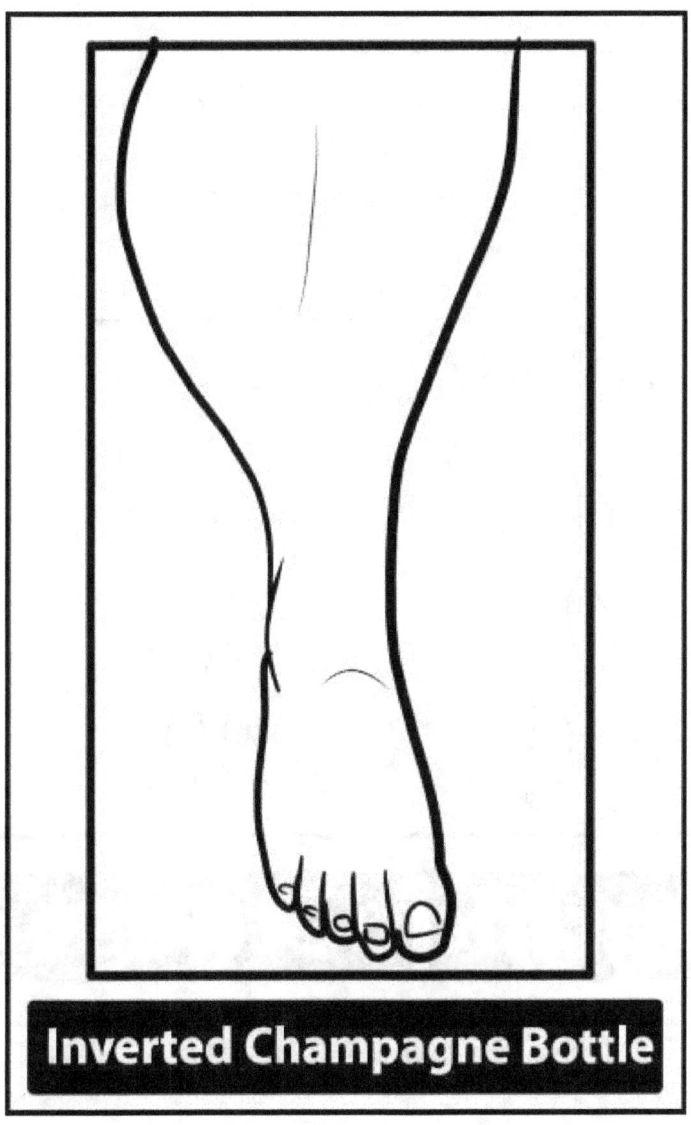

## Venous Vascular Examination

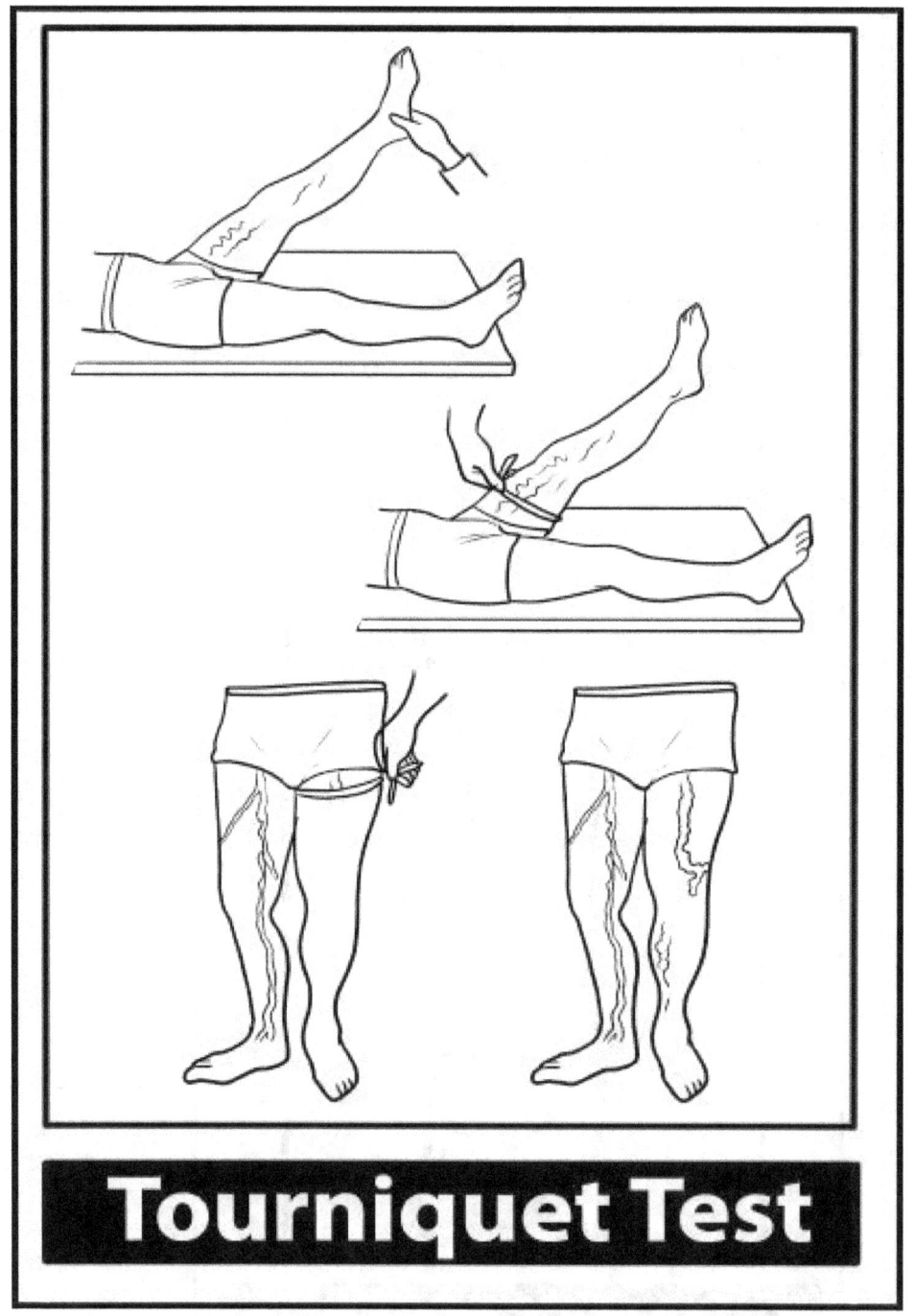

# Arterial Vascular Examination

| | |
|---|---|
| **General** | 1. Wash hands, introduce yourself, get name and age, explain your roles and gain permission<br>2. Supine, legs exposed (wearing shorts)<br>3. Around bed: walking aid, medicine, ECG, insulin<br>4. Patient: pain, Weight |
| **Inspection** | • Swelling<br>• Symmetry<br>• Scars (femoral-popliteal bypass for atherosclerosis in femoral artery, CABG, groin angiogram)<br>• Colour: pale +mottling (acute ischemic limb), black=gangrene dry or wet(moist and **emergency**)<br>• fixed duskiness(non blanchable with pressure = non-viable limb)<br>• Ulcer (between toes, tips of toe, heel, 1 mtp)<br>• Trophic changes in chronic limb ischemia: hair loss, shiny skin, nail dystrophy(thick), muscle atrophy<br>• Amputation |
| **Palpation** | • Temperature (cold: ischemia): back of hands through both legs<br>• Capillary refill: normally less than 2 sec,<br>- check blanchability for dark toe (non blanchable =dead toe)<br>• Pulses:<br>\* if cannot feel pulse do handheld Doppler<br>a) Femoral artery: mid-inguinal point<br>b) Popliteal artery: with flexed knee at 30 degrees and foot in bed feel with tips of fingers<br>\* atherosclerosis commonly affects superficial femoral artery (Hunter canal) so low pulses in popliteal<br><br>**AAA** is associated popliteal aneurysm<br><br>c) Posterior tibial: below medial malleolus<br>d) Dorsalis pedis: lateral to extensor hallucis longus |
| **Auscultate** | - Femoral and abdominal aorta for bruits |
| **Sensation** | - Paresthesia (pin and needles sensation): acute ischemic limb<br>- Same as in neuro examination |

## Arterial Vascular Examination

| | |
|---|---|
| **Special Test** | **Buerger test:**<br>• while supine<br>• Raise leg to 90 degrees (normally no pallor)<br>• In diseased leg pale at 30 (vascular angle)<br>• In severe ischemia vascular angle <20 degrees<br>• Look for venous guttering at this angle<br>• Sit up the patient with both legs dangling from side of bed<br>• From pale to pink > 30 sec = ischemia<br>• From pale to pink to purple red (reactive hyperemia) =chronic ischemia |
| **The End** | **Investigations:**<br>• **blood tests:** glucose, HbA1c, lipid)<br>• **dipstick urine** (microalbuminuria ,glucosuria in DM)<br>• **Ulcer**: Biopsy<br>  - **Discharge for culture**<br>  - **X-ray:** rule out osteomyelitis<br>• ECG(AFIB), Doppler US, CTA, ABPI, arteriography, Exercise treadmill testing<br>• **examine**: Upper limb (pulses + Allen test, adson test, BP)<br>• **Abdomen**: scar +AAA (palpation and auscultation)<br>• **cardiovascular** |

❖ **Neurogenic Claudication:**

- Spinal stenosis
- Pain with walking that radiate from spine to lower limb
- Relieved with bending(flexion) (leaning shopping cart)

▪ **Leriche syndrome:**
- Male
- Aortoiliac occlusion
- Erectile dysfunction
- Femoral pulse absent
- Intermittent claudication buttock, thigh

▪ **Lower Limb ischemia:**

## Arterial Vascular Examination

| Acute ischemia of lower limb | Chronic ischemia of lower limb |
|---|---|
| - **Emboli (acute with only one leg affected**<br>a) Heart: AFib, IE, mural thrombi (MI)<br>b) Arteries: AAA, paradoxical emboli<br>- **Thrombosis of atherosclerosis** (history of intermittent claudication, contralateral limb is affected )(acute on chronic)<br>- **Trauma :**<br>- Fracture<br>- Av fistula<br>- **Compartment syndrome** | - **Atherosclerosis:**<br>- **Risk factors** (DM, smoking, HP, cholesterol, male)<br>- **Buerger's disease:**<br>- Younger than 40 years smoker male |
| - **6 ps:**<br>- Pain(early)<br>- Paraesthesia (early)<br>- Pallor (later cyanosis, fixed mottling)<br>- Pulselessness<br>- Paralysis(late ,non-viable)<br>- Perishingly cold | - Usually in superficial femoral artery (Collateral blood supply at thigh by (profunda femoris)<br>- Critical and non-critical ischemia<br>- **Intermittent claudication and ;location of arteries:**<br>1. **Buttock, thigh pain with ED:** Aortoiliac arteries<br>2. **Calf pain:** femoral, popliteal arteries<br>3. **Forefoot pain :**tibial ,pedal arteries |
| - IV heparin(bolus and infusion)<br>- TPA,streptokinase | - Lifestyle: quit smoking, diet, Exercise (collateral vessels) |
| - Embolectomy :<br>- Fogarty balloon catheter<br>- **Complication**:<br>reperfusion injury:<br><br>a. Edematous painful leg affecting anterior compartment of leg (unable to dorsiflexion)<br>b. Requires fasciotomy<br>- thrombolysis: By catheter<br><br>- Amputation(fixed mottling, paralysis | - Foot care<br>- Risk factors management (HTN, DM)<br>- **Pharmacology:**<br>- Aspirin<br>- **Surgery**:<br>- Bypass graft (Femoro-distal, femoral-popliteal bypass)<br>- Angioplasty and stent<br>- Thromboendarterectomy<br>- Amputation (below knee, above knee)<br>* lumbar sympathectomy for patients unfit for surgery will improve ischemic rest pain, ulceration, gangrene |

## Arterial Vascular Examination

|  |  |
|---|---|
|  |  |

- **ABPI**
  - Doppler US at rest and after treadmill (abi) decreased 20 percent)
    - \>.9 (normal)
    - .5 to .9 (intermittent claudication)
    - .3 to .5 (Rest pain)
    - <.2 (gangrene and ulcer)
  * **False positive** with DM, elderly so use toe brachial index

- **Fontaine classification(PAD)**:(other Rutherford classification)
  I. Asymptomatic
  II. Intermittent claudication.
  III. Rest pain
  IV. tissue loss (ulcer, gangrene)

  * critical limb ischemia: pain at rest, tissue loss (ulceration, gangrene)

- **CRITICAL LIMB ISCHAEMIA:**
  1. Rest pain for more than 2 weeks
     - Worse when legs at the same level of the heart lying at bed
     - Improved with (dependency)dangling the foot at bedside
     - Needs opioid to relieve the pain not OTC analgesia

  2. Tissue loss (ulcer ,gangrene)
  3. ABI<.5

- **AMPUTATION** :Indications (3 **D**'s)
  1. **D**ead: gangrene, Necrotic tissue
  2. **D**angerous: tumor ,wet gangrene, spreading cellulitis
  3. **D**amned nuisance: non-functional limb, severe pain;

## Arterial Vascular Examination

| Ulcer | Ischemic ulcer | Neuropathic ulcer | Venous ulcer |
|---|---|---|---|
| **Causes** | <ul><li>atherosclerosis</li><li>Buerger diseases</li><li>vasculitis</li></ul> | <ul><li>Unknown</li><li>DM</li></ul> | <ul><li>CVI*May become Marjolin's ulcer(SCC)</li></ul> |
| **Leg/foot** | <ul><li>Trophic changes (CLI)</li><li>Pulseless</li></ul> | <ul><li>Leg charcot joint</li><li>Hammer claw</li><li>Claw toe</li><li>Callus</li><li>Decreased sensation</li><li>warm, well perfused</li></ul> | <ul><li>Same features in CVI</li></ul> |
| **Site** | <ul><li>**pressure areas:**<br>- Between and tips of toe, heel, lateral malleolus</li></ul> | <ul><li>**Plantar surface:** metatarsal head (first)</li><li>Pressure area( heel)</li></ul> | <ul><li>Gaiter area (medial side)</li></ul> |
| **Size** | <ul><li>Small</li></ul> | <ul><li>Small</li></ul> | <ul><li>Large</li></ul> |
| **Border and edge** | <ul><li>Round regular punched out edge</li></ul> | <ul><li>Regular callus border punched-out edge</li></ul> | <ul><li>Irregular border and sloping edges</li><li>Exudate</li></ul> |
| **Other** | <ul><li>Dry</li><li>Painful</li><li>Yellow base(slough)</li></ul> | <ul><li>Painless</li></ul> | <ul><li>Painless unless infected</li><li>granulated base(floor)</li></ul> |

## Arterial Vascular Examination

- **DD:**
  - Pyoderma gangrenosum: IBD/RA
  - Rodent ulcer (BCC): face due sun damage
  - Martorell ulcer: HTN
  - Marjolin's ulcer(SCC)

- **AAA:**
  - Mostly infrarenal
  - Localized dilation >3cms
  - Presentation: asymptomatic , back pain , hypotension
  - Detected by abdominal ultrasound
  - Indications for treatment:
1. Symptomatic
2. Asymptomatic >5.5cm , or growing >1cm/ yearly

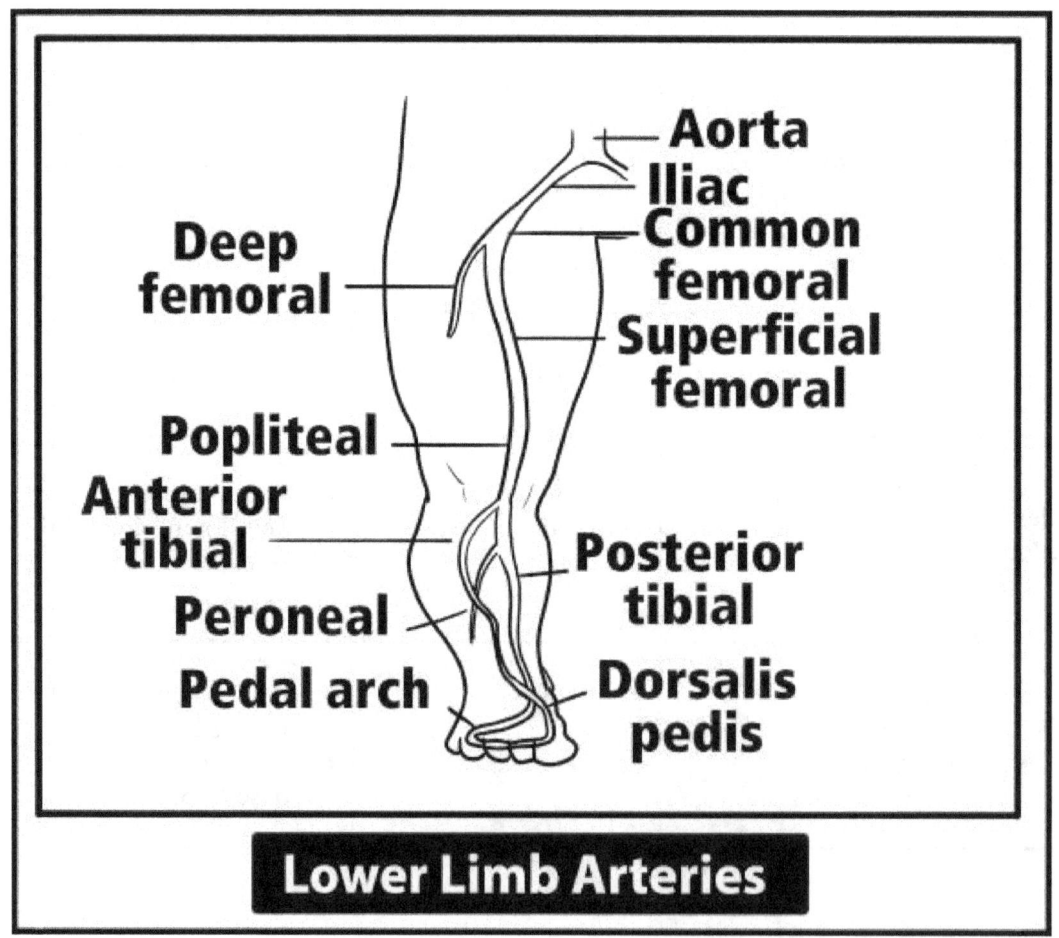

## Arterial Vascular Examination

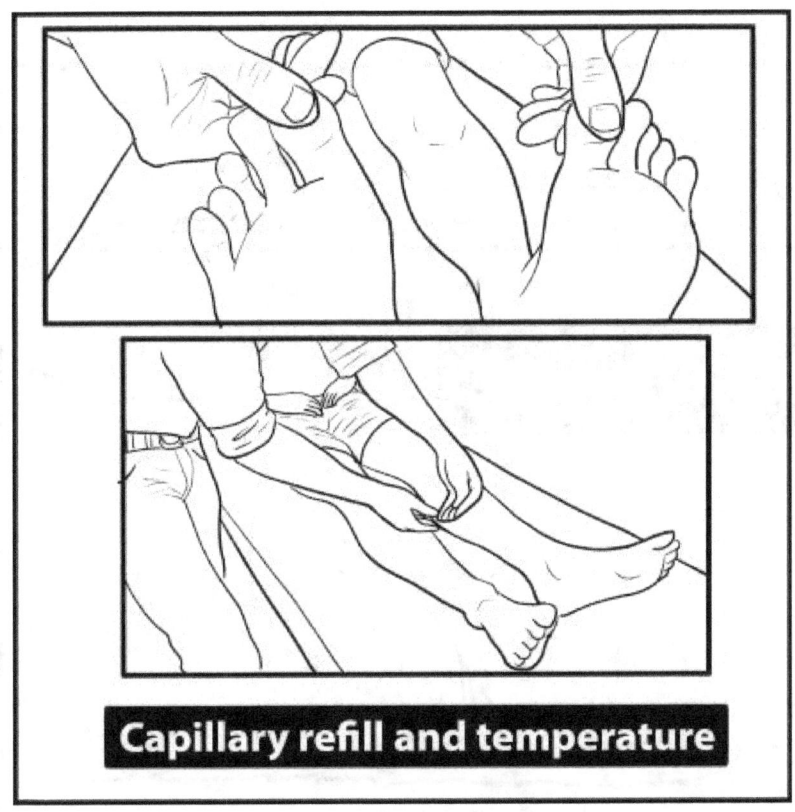

**Capillary refill and temperature**

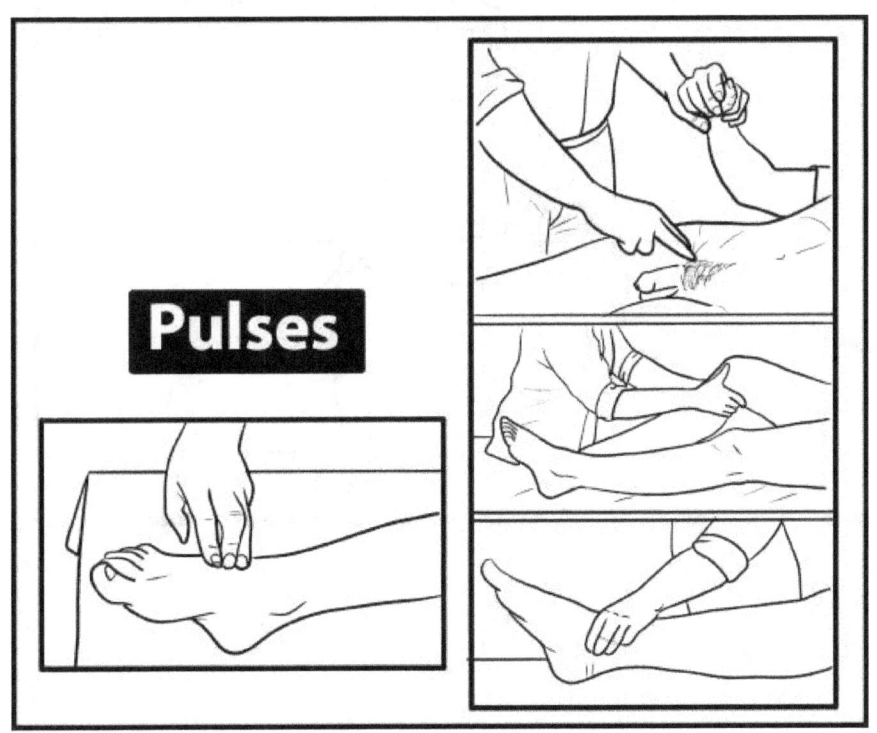

**Pulses**

# Arterial Vascular Examination

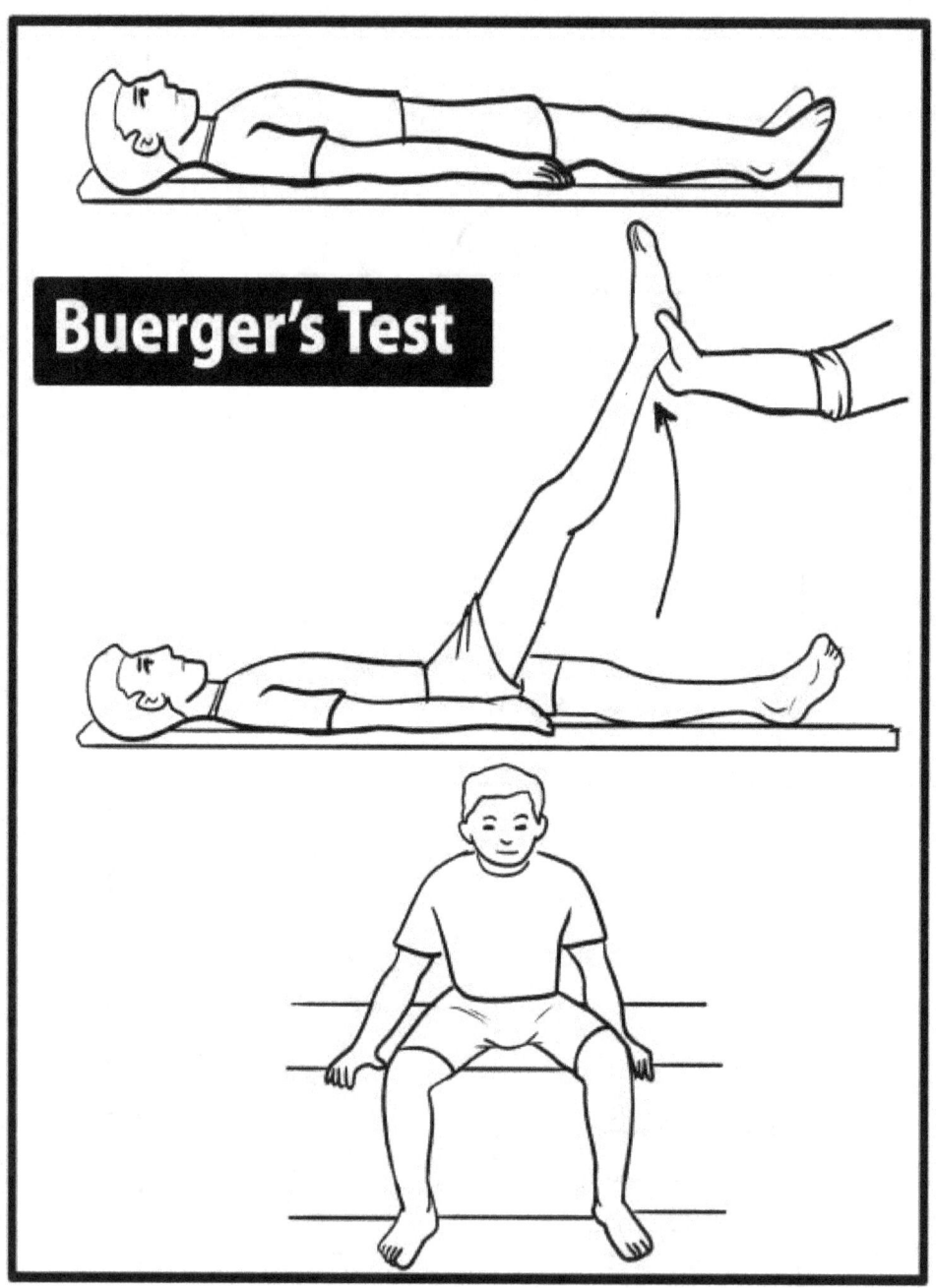

## Shoulder Examination

| | |
|---|---|
| **General** | 1. Wash hands, introduce yourself, get name and age, explain your role out pain and gain permission<br>2. Standing, chest exposed (no shirt)<br>3. Around bed (walking aid, medicine)<br>4. Patient (BMI, age, pain, fever, Septic arthritis and PMR) |
| **Inspection** | • **Anteriorly, laterally, posteriorly**<br>- Swelling, redness (Inflammation: RA SA, gout, tendonitis, bursitis (subacromial))<br>- Ecchymosis (trauma, tendon rupture)<br>- Asymmetry<br>- Atrophy:<br>a. deltoid flattens (axillary N palsy due anterior dislocation, humeral surgical neck fracture))<br>b. supraspinous and infraspinous atrophy (prominence of spine of scapula) due Rotator muscle tear<br>- Posture: scoliosis (one shoulder elevated)<br>- Scars (shoulder replacement, arthroscopy)<br>- Fracture(clavicle)<br>- Popeye sign during flexion (bicipital tendon rupture)<br>- Wall push up test: (winged scapula due long thoracic N in stab wound, dissection of axillary lymph)<br>    * scapular dyskinesis causes impingement syndrome |
| **Palpation** | - Temperature(inflammation): back of hand anterior and posterior of shoulder<br>- Palpate: for tenderness watch face (inflammation), swelling<br>- SCJ-clavicle-ACJ -acromion-coracoid process (2cm inferior and medial to the clavicular tip)- spine of scapula, borders of scapula<br>- head of humerus(bursitis)<br>- bicipital groove (Bicipital tendinitis) |
| **Movements** | • **Active vs Passive**<br>- place hand over shoulder during passive movement (crepitus)<br>- Notice pain, ROM<br>• Flexion 180°<br>• Extension 60°<br>• Abduction 180°: supraspinatus 15, deltoid 15-90, serratus anterior + deltoid 90-180 |

## Shoulder Examination

|  | *See scapula comment on scapulohumeral rhythm on abduction scapula (inferior angle) 1:2 humeral<br><br>- Adduction<br>- External rotation 90°<br>- Internal rotation 90° |
|---|---|
| **Special Tests** | - **Hawkin Test:**<br>  - Patient standing<br>  - Passively flex both Shoulder and elbow flexed at 90°<br>  - Internally rotate the shoulder<br>  - **Pain** =impingement syndrome<br><br>- **Neer Test:**<br>  - Position yourself behind Pt<br>  - Stabilize the scapula with one of your hand<br>  - With other hand internally rotate Pt arm ,then full flex his arm<br>  - Pain =  impingement syndrome<br><br>- **Empty can Test (Jobe):**<br>  - Patient standing<br>  - Shoulder flexed 90°<br>  - Elbow extended<br>  - Shoulder Abducted 30°<br>  - Shoulder Internally rotated (thumb downward)<br>  - Ask patient to raise arms while you are resisting (downward pressure)<br>  - **Pain**=supraspinatus defect<br><br>- **Infraspinatus and Teres Minor Test:**<br>  - Elbow tucked and flexed at 90°<br>  - Ask patient to externally rotate shoulder while you are resisting<br><br>- **Gerber Test (subscapularis)**<br>  - Dorsum of hand rest on the back<br>  - Ask patient to left off hand (internal rotation) while you are resisting<br><br>- **Apprehension Test (crank):**<br>  - Lying flat<br>  - Passively abduct shoulder and flex elbow at 90°<br>  - Externally rotated shoulder<br>  - **Pain**=shoulder instability |

## Shoulder Examination

|  |  |
|---|---|
|  | • **Cross-Body Adduction for AC joint injury :**<br>- Passively elevate Pt arm to 90 degrees and abduct it across the body |
| **The End** | - Upper limb neurological examination<br>- spurling test (cervical radiculopathy), Lhermitte sign (cervical myelopathy+finger escape sign)<br>- Vascular examination<br>- Thoracic outlet syndrome (adson test)<br>- X-ray, MRI<br>- ESR |

❖ **RC muscles:**
- SITS
- **Supraspinatus:** abduction
- **Infraspinatus and teres minor:** external rotation
- **Subscapularis:** internal rotation

### 1. Impingement Syndrome:

compression of rotator cuff tendons (supraspinatus mostly) & bursa (subacromial) between humeral head and acromion causing, rotator cuff tendonitis & subarachnoid bursitis.

- **Risk Factors:**
- Osteophyte(elderly)
- overhead activities(young)

- **Clinical Features:**
- Dull pain in anterolateral shoulder
- Worsen by overhead activities, at night (lying on diseased side)
- Painful arc test: pain during abduction(60-120 degrees)
- positive Neer impingement test & Hawkins test
- Decreased ROM

- **Investigation:**
- MRI

- **Treatment:**
1. Physiotherapy
2. NSAIDS
3. Subacromial injection(steroid)
4. Arthroscopic subacromial decompression (ASD)

## Shoulder Examination

### 2. Frozen shoulder (adhesive capsulitis):

- **Risk Factors:**
  - DM, thyroid(hyperthyroidism), immobilization, female

- **Clinical Features**
  - restriction ROM in all motions (active and passive) and pain
  * **early loss of external rotation movement**

- **Stages:**
  - duration around **18** months
  a. **Freezing:** pain
  b. **Frozen:** stiffness
  c. **Thawing:** gradually back to normal

- **Investigations:**
  - MRI

- **Treatment**
  - NSAID
  - physiotherapy
  - Intra-articular injection(steroid)
  - Surgery

### 3. Polymyalgia Rheumatica:
- Old female

- **Clinical Features:**
  - Bilateral Pain and stiffness in proximal muscle (shoulder, hips) that improved with exercise and worsen with rest
  - Systemic symptoms (fever, Weight loss)
  - Seen in temporal arteritis

  - High ESR
  - Treated by steroid

- **Other drugs causes myopathy is :**
  1. Statin
  2. glucocorticoid

# Shoulder Examination

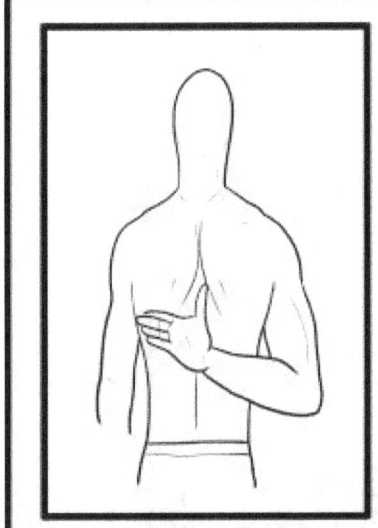

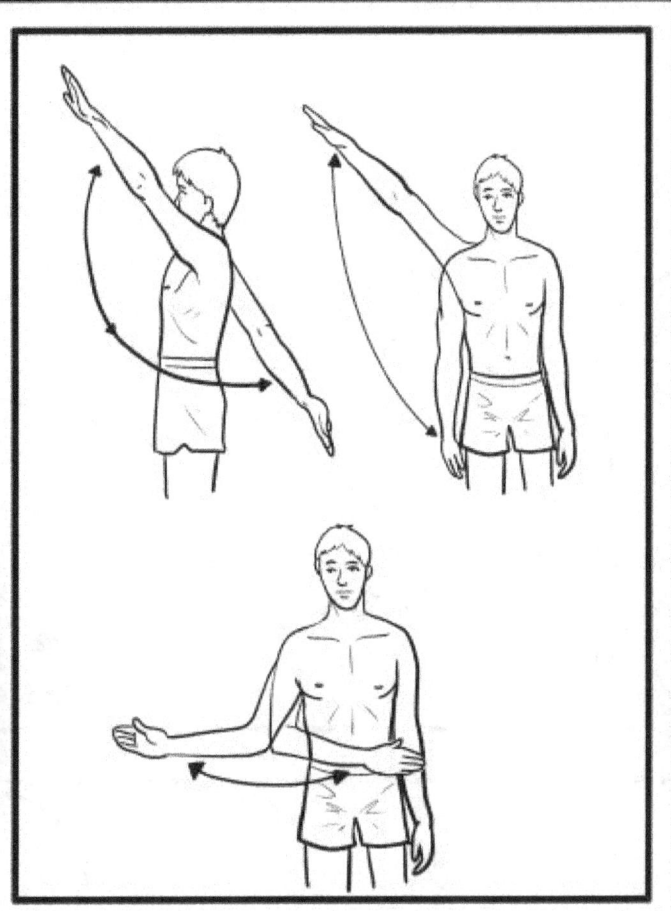

**Movements:**
- abduction
- adduction
- external
- internal rotations

## Shoulder Examination

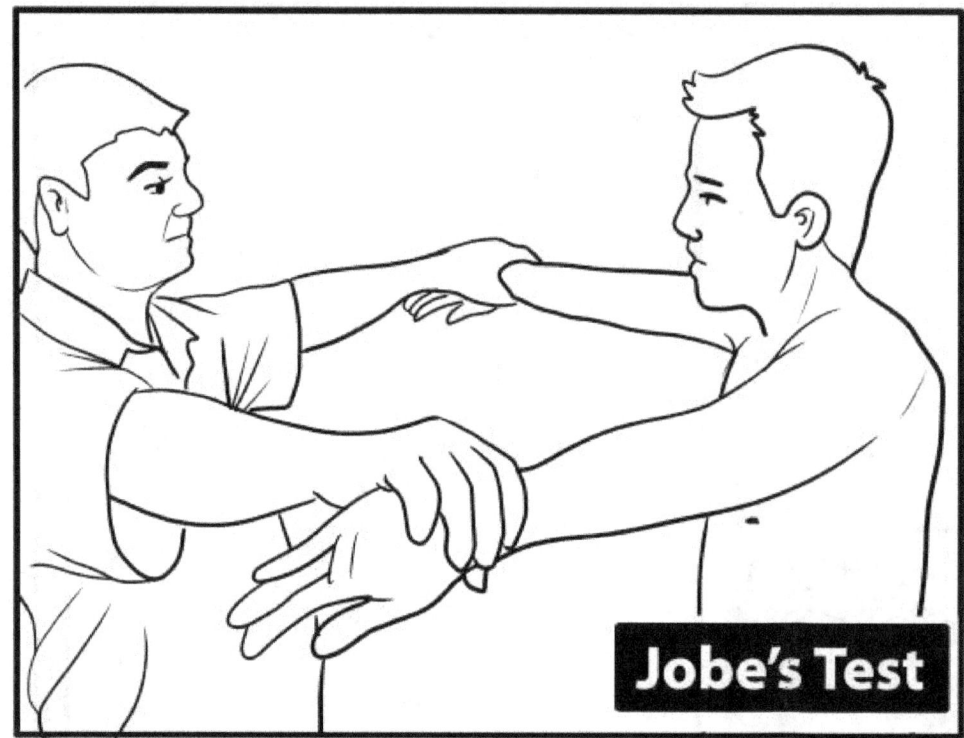

Jobe's Test

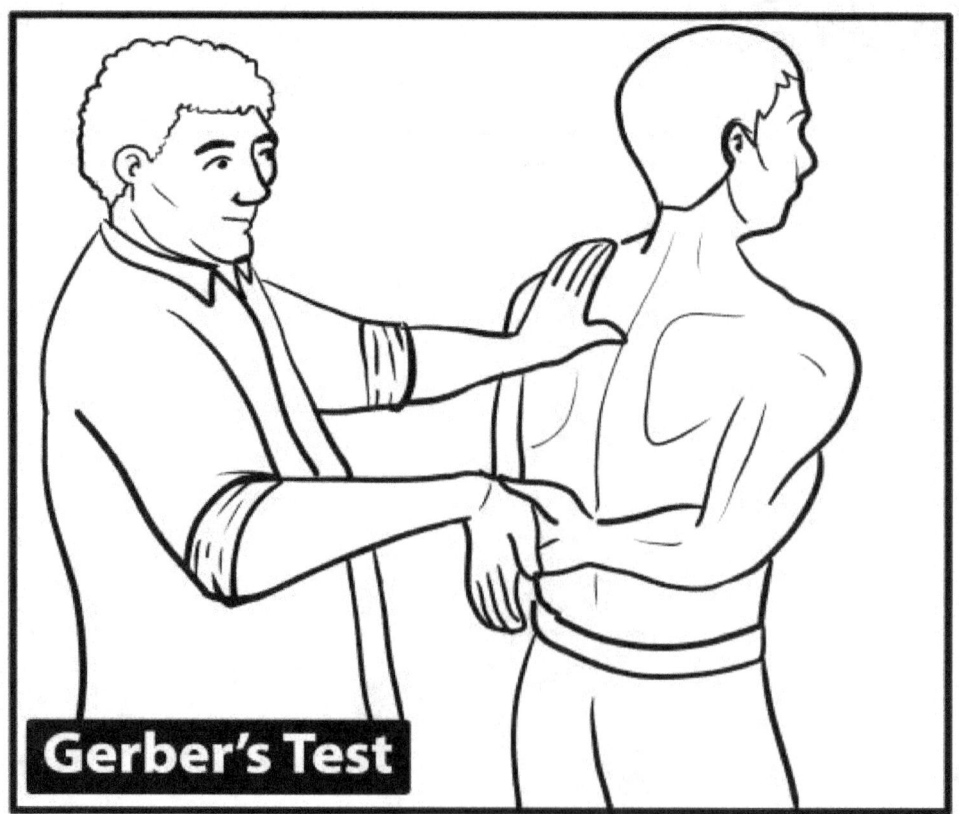

Gerber's Test

# Shoulder Examination

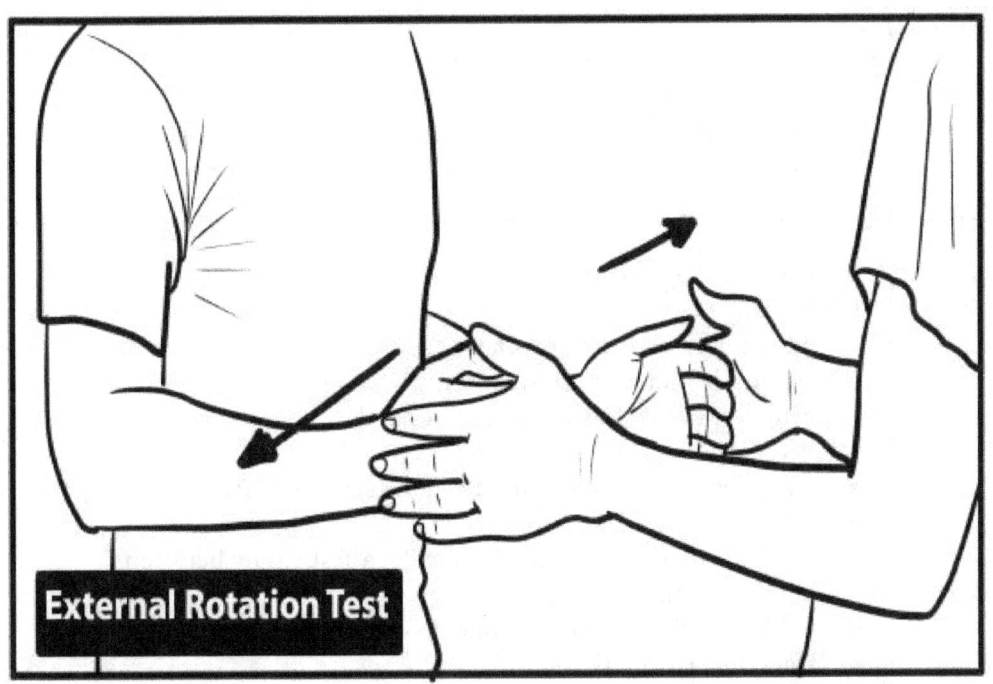

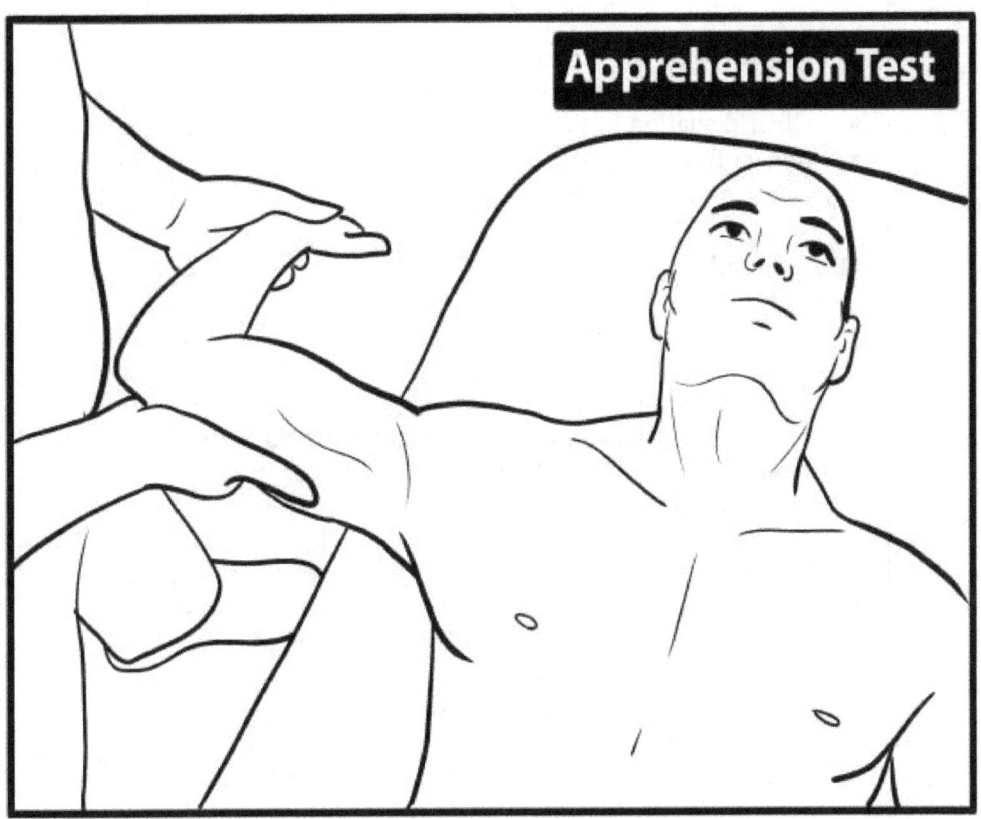

## Hand Examination

| | |
|---|---|
| **General** | 1. Wash hands, introduce yourself, get name and age, explain your roles and gain permission<br>2. Arms exposed, till the elbow patient seated comfortably, hands over pillow |
| **Inspection** | ❖ **Compare for symmetry:**<br>1. **Nails:**<br>• pitting, Onycholysis (psoriatic arthritis)<br>• splinter hemorrhage (RA, vasculitis)<br>2. **Fingers, hand, wrist**: dorsum of hands<br>a) **Swelling:**<br>• OA (Heberden's nodes at DIP, bouchard's at PIP)<br>• rheumatoid nodule<br>• MCP synovitis (Ask patient to make a fest valley between knuckles will be lost)<br>• Diffuse (infection, compartment syndrome)<br>• Dactylitis (psoriatic arthritis)<br>• **Other:** Garrod's pads (dupuytren contracture)<br><br>b) **Deviation:**<br>• A Radial deviation of wrist (RA)<br>• Ulnar deviation of fingers (RA)<br>• fingers fractures (ask to flex fingers see any malrotation of fingers which normally point to scaphoid)<br><br>c) **Deformity:**<br>▪ **RA**:<br>- Swan neck (hyperextension of DIP + flexion of PIP)<br>- Boutine (hyperextension of PIP + flexion of DIP)<br>- Z-shaped thumb<br>- Vaughan-Jackson syndrome (extensor tendon rupture)<br>- Prominent ulnar styloid<br><br>▪ **Others**<br>• Mallet finger (Dip flexion): move passively but not actively<br>• Flexion deformity :partial claw hands(medial fingers) due ulnar n palsy ,complete claw hand klumpke syndrome<br>• dinner fork deformity (colles fracture): due to fall on an outstretched hand in osteoporosis elderly female Opposite to smith fracture<br>3. **Interosseous muscle atrophy(back of hand):** (RA, ulnar palsy, T1 lesion especially first web)<br><br>- **Color:** |

## Hand Examination

|  |  |
|---|---|
|  | <ul><li>Erythema(cellulitis)</li><li>Raynaud's disease (SLE, RA)</li></ul>4. palmer side:<ul><li>Thenar atrophy (median nerve palsy in carpal tunnel syndrome</li><li>Hypothenar (ulnar nerve)</li><li>Dupuytren's contracture</li><li>Z shaped scar for dupuytren surgery</li><li>Palmar erythema (RA)</li><li>Scars (carpal tunnel syndrome, Dermofasciectomy scars for Dupuytren's contracture)</li></ul>5. Elbow (psoriatic plaques, Rheumatoid nodules)<br>6. Ear, scalp (gouty tophi, psoriatic plaques) |
| **Palpation** | 1. Temperature with back of your hands over the dorsum of patient hand (inflammation)<br>2. Palpate:<br>- swelling<br>a) firm bony (OA)<br>b) spongy (synovitis ,ganglion ,nodules)<br>- tenderness (watch patient face)<br>- start with:<br>  1. elbow(rheumatoid nodules<br>  2. wrist<br>- palpate distal radius and ulna using your two thumbs press laterally to medially.<br>* tenderness in distal radius (colles fracture)<br>* tenderness in radial styloid around extensor pollicis longus and abductor pollicis longus (de quervain tenosynovitis)<br>* tenderness in snuff box (scaphoid fracture)<br>- palpate each MCP or squeeze MCP between your thumb and fingers<br>- Palpate PIP, DIP with box technique (joint is palpated by four fingers simultaneously)<br>- palpate palm:<br>*   Thickness of palmar fascia (Dupuytren's contracture)<br>* Muscle mass(atrophy)<br>* Nodules on flexor tendon (trigger finger seen in DM) |
|  | ▪ **Restrictive ROM**: arthritis, tenosynovitis, Dupuytren's contracture |

# Hand Examination

| | |
|---|---|
| **Movements** <br> active vs passive | 1. **Wrist**: <br> • Flexion: prayer sign <br> • Extension: Reverse pray sign <br> • Adduction(radial) <br> • abduction(ulnar) <br> 2. **Fingers** <br> • Flexion, Extension <br> • Notice any (trigger fingers) inability to fully extend finger from fully flexed fingers <br> • Abduction, adduction <br> 3. **Thumb**: <br> • Flexion, Extension <br> • Abduction, Adduction <br> • Opposition |
| **Vascular and neurological** | • **Vascular**: <br>   - capillary refill, radial pulse, ulnar pulse, Allen's test <br><br> ➤ **Neurological exam :** <br>   - Quick screen :Use 'Paper – scissors – stone <br>   - Look at the image below <br><br> • **Motor**: while you are resisting <br>   - Thumb abduction (median nerve) <br>   - fingers extension (radial nerve) <br>   - Fingers abduction (ulnar nerve) <br><br> • **Sensory**: <br>   - cotton, pin tip (closed eye) <br>   - Pulp index finger (median nerve) <br>   - Fifth finger (ulnar) <br>   - Dorsal web space thumb (radial) <br><br> • **Function :** <br>   - Undo button , Power grip(squeeze your fingers),pick up a coin |
| **Special Tests** | 1. Finkelstein test for de quervain tenosynovitis <br>   - ask to make a fist with thumb inside fist <br>   - stabilizing the forearm and ulnarly deviate the fist <br>   - positive sign if pain in radial styloid <br><br> 2. Carpal tunnel syndrome tests by <br> a) **Tinel sign** <br>   - tap over flexor retinaculum |

## Hand Examination

|  |  |
|---|---|
| | b) **Phalen sign**<br>- reverse prayer signs for 60 sec<br>c) **Durkan's test**<br>- Positive sign if pins and needles sensations in median nerve disruptive<br><br>3. Ulnar nerve palsy<br>- **Froment's sign:**<br>- Ask the Pt to hold a paper between his thumb and Radial side of his index and not to let it go<br>- Now pull the paper with your hand<br>- Positive if flexion at thumb IP<br><br>- **Wartenberg's sign:**<br>- Ask Pt to abduct his extended fingers<br>- Positive if unopposed abduction of little finger<br><br>- **Tabletop test:**<br>- Ask Pt to put his palmer side of his hand on a table<br>- Positive if unable to fully lay his hand on the table |
| The End | - **To complete**<br>- Elbow, shoulder exam and upper neuro examinations needed to be done |

### ❖ Median N
- **Motor:**
- LOAF muscles
- Lateral two lumbricals
- Opponens pollicis
- Abductor pollicis brevis
- Flexor pollicis brevis

| Carpal Tunnel Syndrome | Dupuytren Contracture |
|---|---|

## Hand Examination

|  | (median N compression) |  |
|---|---|---|
| **Present as** | - Numbness and tingling in lateral fingers<br>- Awaken Pt from sleep<br>- Improve with shaking out the hand<br>* sensory part of median nerve is spared<br>* motor part is affected (thenar atrophy) | - Painless palmar nodules<br>- Thickened palmar fascia flexed 4th and 5th finger and inability to extend them |
| **Causes** | - pregnancy<br>- RA<br>- Hypothyroidism<br>- Lipoma<br>- Amyloid<br>- Idiopathic<br>- Lunate dislocation | - Family history<br>- DM<br>- Alcohol<br>- Alcoholic cirrhosis |
| **Investigation** | - EMG<br>- nerve conduction study | |
| **Managed** | - NSAIDS, splints<br>- Steroid injections<br>- Carpal tunnel release | - Collagenase, steroid injection<br>- Fasciectomy or needle fasciotomy |

## Hand Examination

### ❖ Rheumatoid arthritis

| | |
|---|---|
| **Present in** | • Female & genetic (HLA-DRA4) |
| **Features** | • **Symmetrical polyarthritis for more than 6 weeks**<br>• (tender, swollen, painful) of peripheral joints:<br>  - Wrist and hands(PIP+MCP)<br>  - Feet, ankle, knees<br><br>• Present as multiple joints pain and stiffness for more >1 hr in morning<br>  - Worsen with rest<br>  - Improve with exercises<br>  - Weight loss, fever |
| **Extra-articular manifestations** | • **Eye**: Sjögren syndrome, Scleritis, anterior uveitis (painful red eye)<br>• **Thorax**: pericarditis, Aortitis (aortic reg), pleural effusion, interstitial lung disease (progressive dyspnea, cor pulmonale), Bronchiolitis obliterans organizing pneumonia<br>• **Renal**: nephrotic syndrome due Amyloidosis<br>• **Musculoskeletal:**<br>  - Protrusio acetabuli(hip)<br>  - Synovial cysts (baker's cyst)<br>  - Atlantoaxial subluxation (Cervical myelopathy): do cervical x ray before intubation or general anesthesia<br>  - vasculitis: Mononeuritis multiplex(foot drop)<br>  - skin ulcer<br>**Anaemia**: due<br><br>  a. Drug (NSAID(low MCV) methotrexate(high MCV)<br>  b. Felty syndrome<br>  c. Anemia of chronic diseases<br><br>-vision:<br><br>  a. Episcleritis<br>  b. Sjögren syndrome<br>- **neurological**:<br><br>  a. Peripheral neuropathy(sensory<br>  b. Carpal tunnel syndrome |

# Hand Examination

|  |  |
|---|---|
|  | c. Mononeuritis multiplex (motor )<br>d. Cervical subluxation<br><br>- **syndromes:**<br><br>    - Caplan syndrome (pneumoconiosis)<br>    - Felty syndrome (Splenomegaly and granulocytopenia) |
| **Investigate** | - **Lab:**<br>    - Anti ccp (specific), RF(sensitive)<br>    - ESR+CRP<br>    - Normocytic anemia<br>- **Imaging**: X ray<br>    - Soft tissue swelling<br>    - Juxta-articular osteoporosis<br>    - Joint space narrowing and erosions especially Ulnar styloid |
| **Management** | - **Smoking cessation**<br>- **Symptomatic relief:**<br>    - Nsaid(not for PUD, CRF<br>    - Steroid(prednisone)<br><br>- **DMARDs:**<br>a) Methotrexate<br>  - Measure LFT and stop alcohol to avoid Hepatotoxicity<br>  - Measure creatinine to avoid nephrotoxicity<br>  - Bone marrow suppression ,mouth ulcer<br>  - Contradicted during pregnancy<br>* Folate helps in minimizing the complication<br><br>b) Sulfasalazine<br>c) Leflunomide<br>d) Hydroxychloroquine sulfate: check eye yearly (vision loss)<br><br>- **Biologic agents:**<br>1. Tnf inhibitor: infliximab: chest x ray and tuberculin test for TB reactivation<br>2. Abatacept<br>3. Rituximab<br><br>- **Surgical treatment: for severe pain and functional disability**<br>  - Synovectomy, Arthrodesis, joint replacement.<br>  - DAS28: to evaluate disease activity: number of tender & |

## Hand Examination

|   |   |
|---|---|
|   | swollen joints, ESR, patient global health<br>- ACR-EULAR: classification criteria for RA: number of joints, serology (RF, Anti CCP) ,duration (more than 6 weeks), Acute Phase Reactants(ESR+CRP) |

### ❖ Sjögren Syndrome:

- **Autoimmune disease exocrine glands**
- **Present as :**
a. **Sicca symptoms:**
- Keratoconjunctivitis sicca (dry eye)
- Xerostomia (dry mouth)
- Dyspareunia (dry vaigina)
b. **salivary gland enlargement (enlarged parotid gland)**
c. **a B-cell lymphoma**
- **Investigation:**
- Anti Ro/SSA and La/SSB (mom with these AB might give a birth for an infant with heart block)
- ANA (+)
- RF (+)
- lip biopsy (inflammatory infiltrate)

- **Management:**
- Artificial tears
- Pilocarpine

### ❖ Psoriatic arthritis

- **Clinical features:**
a. **Skin**: itchy scaly silvery plaque on extensor surfaces elbows, knees, scalp
b. **Joints involvement pattern:**
- Arthritis of DIP (Pencil-in-cup deformity)
- Asymmetric oligoarticular
- Symmetrical RA like
- Arthritis mutilans (opera glass hand)
- Axial involvement(spine and sacroiliac joint)

- **Treatment**
- NSAID
- UV light
- DMARDs and biological agent for arthritis

### ❖ Systemic Lupus Erythematosus:

## Hand Examination

- **Clinical features :** 4 or more of these features are needed to confirm the diagnosis

1. **Face :**
   - malar ("butterfly") rash: spares nasolabial folds
   - Photosensitivity
   - oral ulcers
   - neurological(stroke ,seizure)

2. **Thorax and abdomen :**
   - Serositis (pleural and pericardial effusion )
   - Diffuse alveolar hemorrhage
   - Kidney(glomerulonephritis)

3. **Extremities:**
   - hematological(pancytopenia)
   - antiphospholipid syndrome
   - Arthritis
   - discoid rash

\* cardiovascular disease is the usually the cause of death

- **Investigations:**
- ANA (sensitive)
- Anti dsDNA antibody (specific)
- Low c3 ,c4 (acute flare up)
- Anti-Smith antibody (specific)
- Anti-histone antibody(drug-induced lupus)

- **Management**
- Sun cream
- Arthritis: NSAIDs ,Hydroxychloroquine ,Steroid

❖ **Scleroderma**

|  | Limited Cutaneous | Diffuse scleroderma |
|---|---|---|
| **Features** | <ul><li>ANA</li><li>Anticentromere antibodies</li><li>Pulmonary hypertension</li><li>CREST syndrome:</li><li>Calcinosis</li><li>Raynaud's phenomenon: cold cause fingers turn white then blue</li><li>Esophageal dysmotility</li></ul> | <ul><li>ANA</li><li>Anti–Scl-70 antibodies</li><li>GERD</li><li>Interstitial lung disease</li><li>Renal crisis (hypertension)</li><li>Malabsorption (bacterial overgrowth_</li></ul> |

## Hand Examination

| | | |
|---|---|---|
| | • Sclerodactyly<br>• telangiectasia | |
| **Management** | • Avoid cold<br>• Calcium blocker (Raynaud phenomenon)<br>• pulmonary hypertension (oxygen ,endothelin receptor antagonist, phosphodiesterase 5 inhibitor) | • Renal : acei<br>• GERD:PPI<br>• Bacterial overgrowth: antibiotic<br>• Interstitial fibrosis:<br>• Cyclophosphamide |

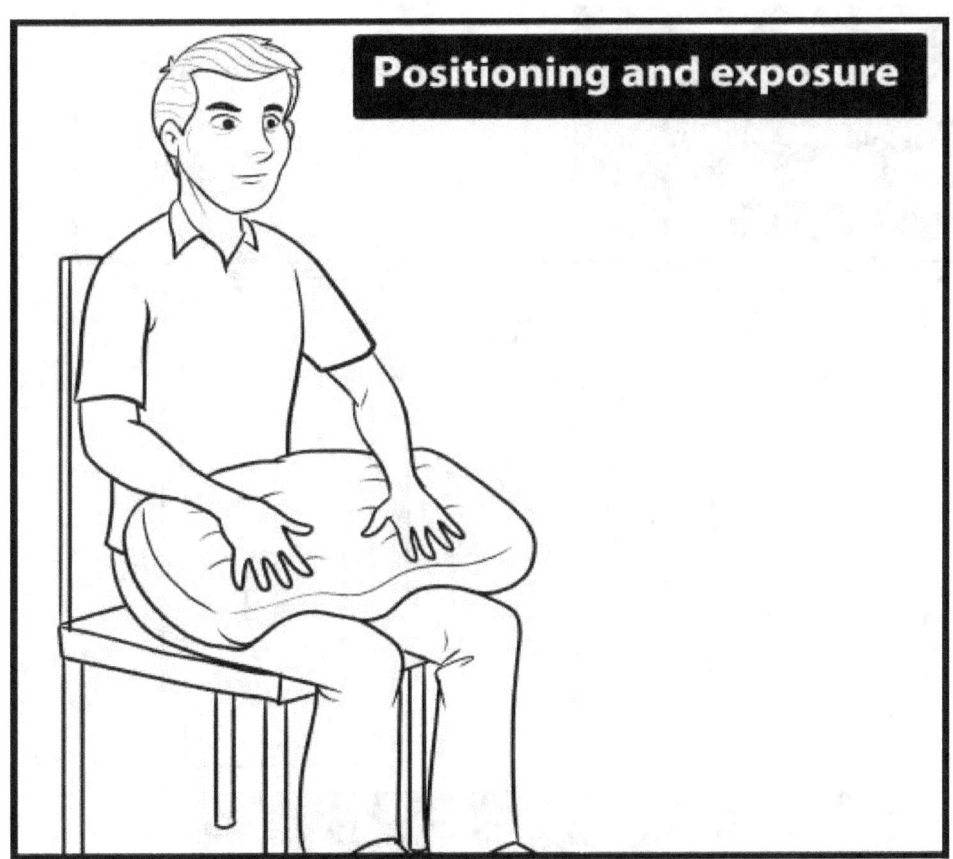

# Hand Examination

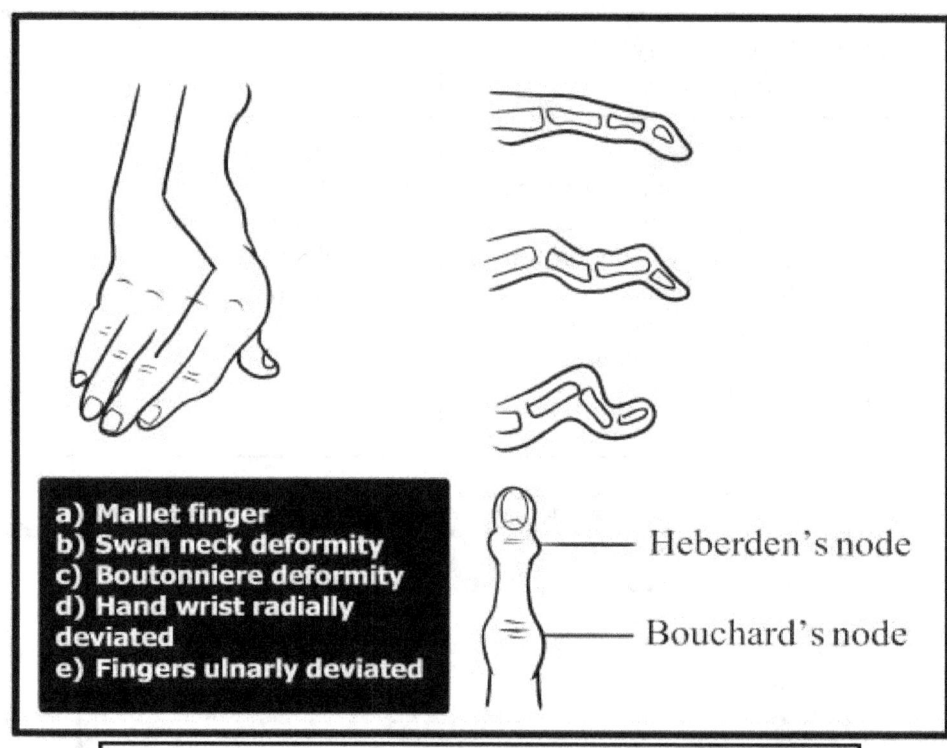

a) Mallet finger
b) Swan neck deformity
c) Boutonniere deformity
d) Hand wrist radially deviated
e) Fingers ulnarly deviated

Heberden's node
Bouchard's node

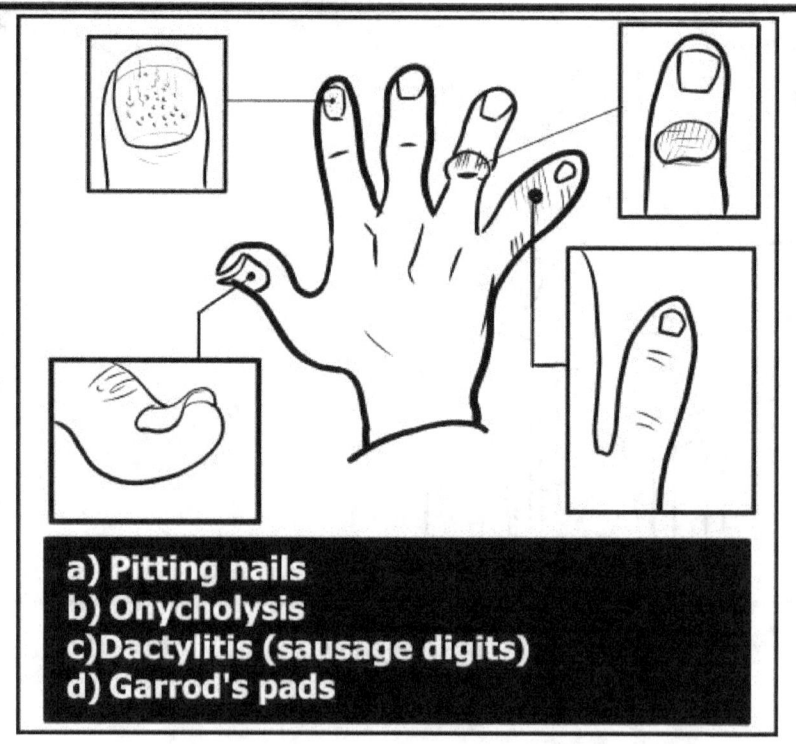

a) Pitting nails
b) Onycholysis
c) Dactylitis (sausage digits)
d) Garrod's pads

## Hand Examination

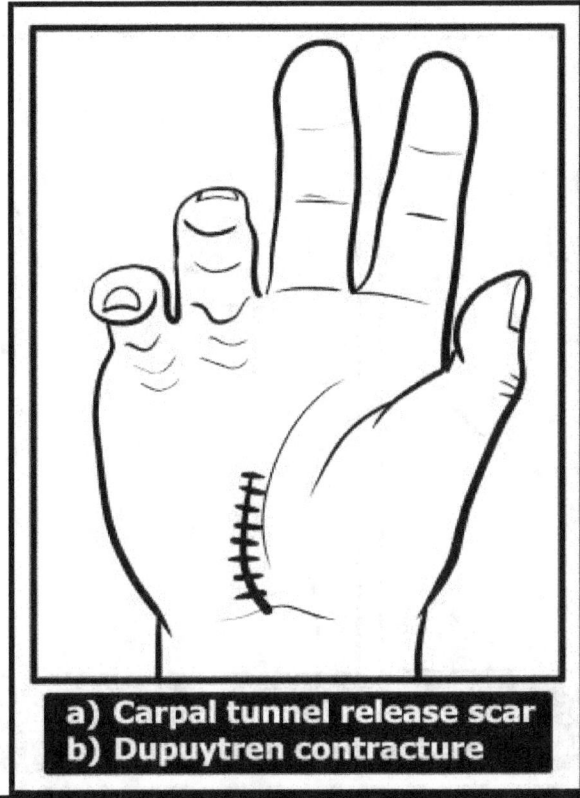

a) Carpal tunnel release scar
b) Dupuytren contracture

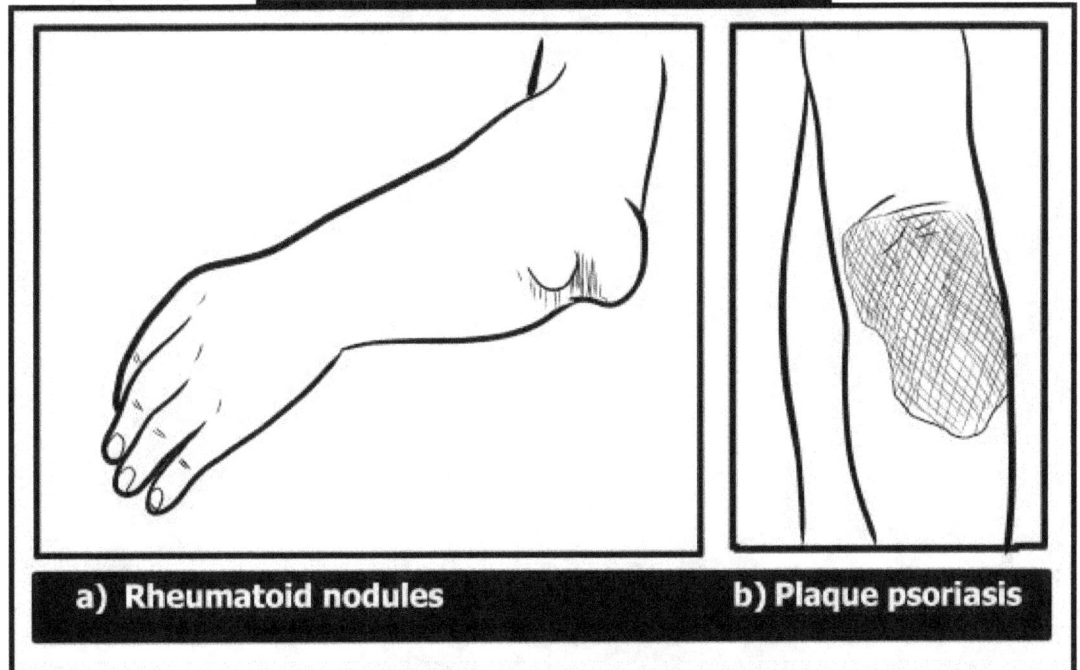

a) Rheumatoid nodules
b) Plaque psoriasis

# Hand Examination

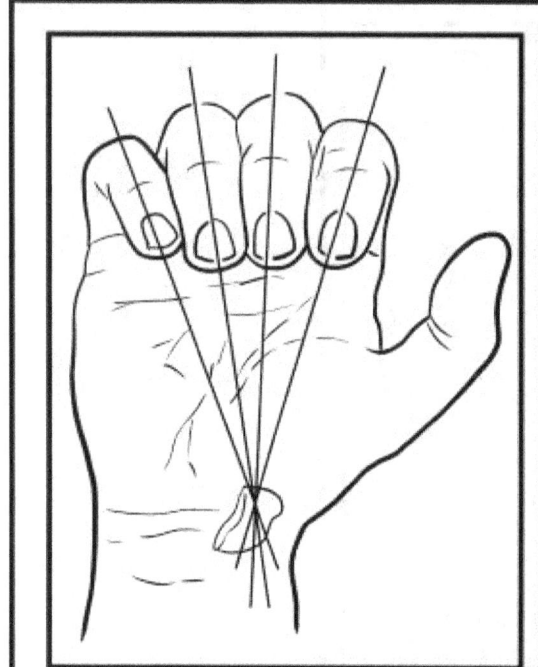 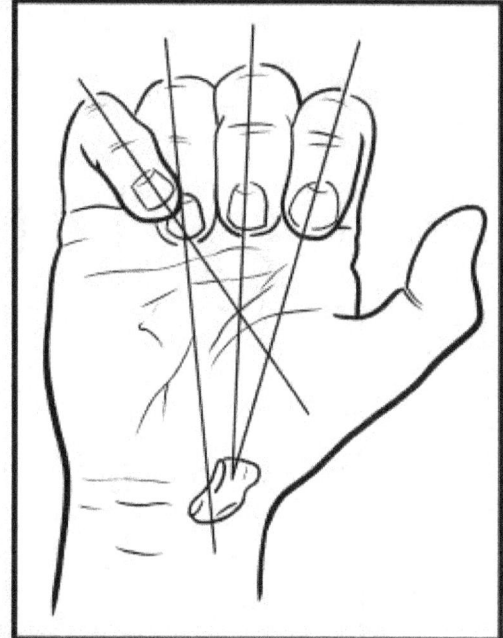

**Malrotation of fingers which normally point to scaphoid (little finger is fractured here)**

# Hand Examination

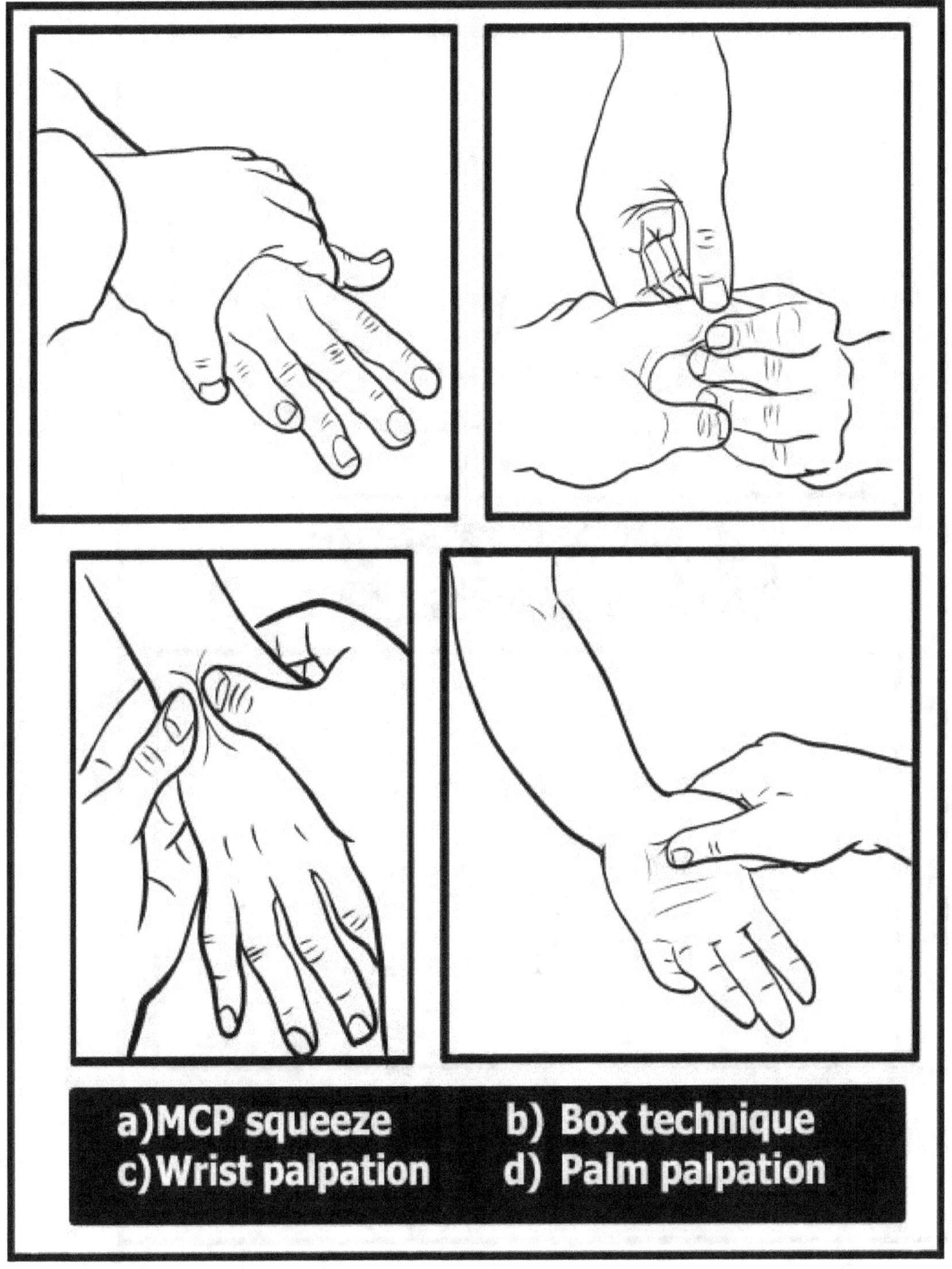

a) MCP squeeze    b) Box technique
c) Wrist palpation    d) Palm palpation

# Hand Examination

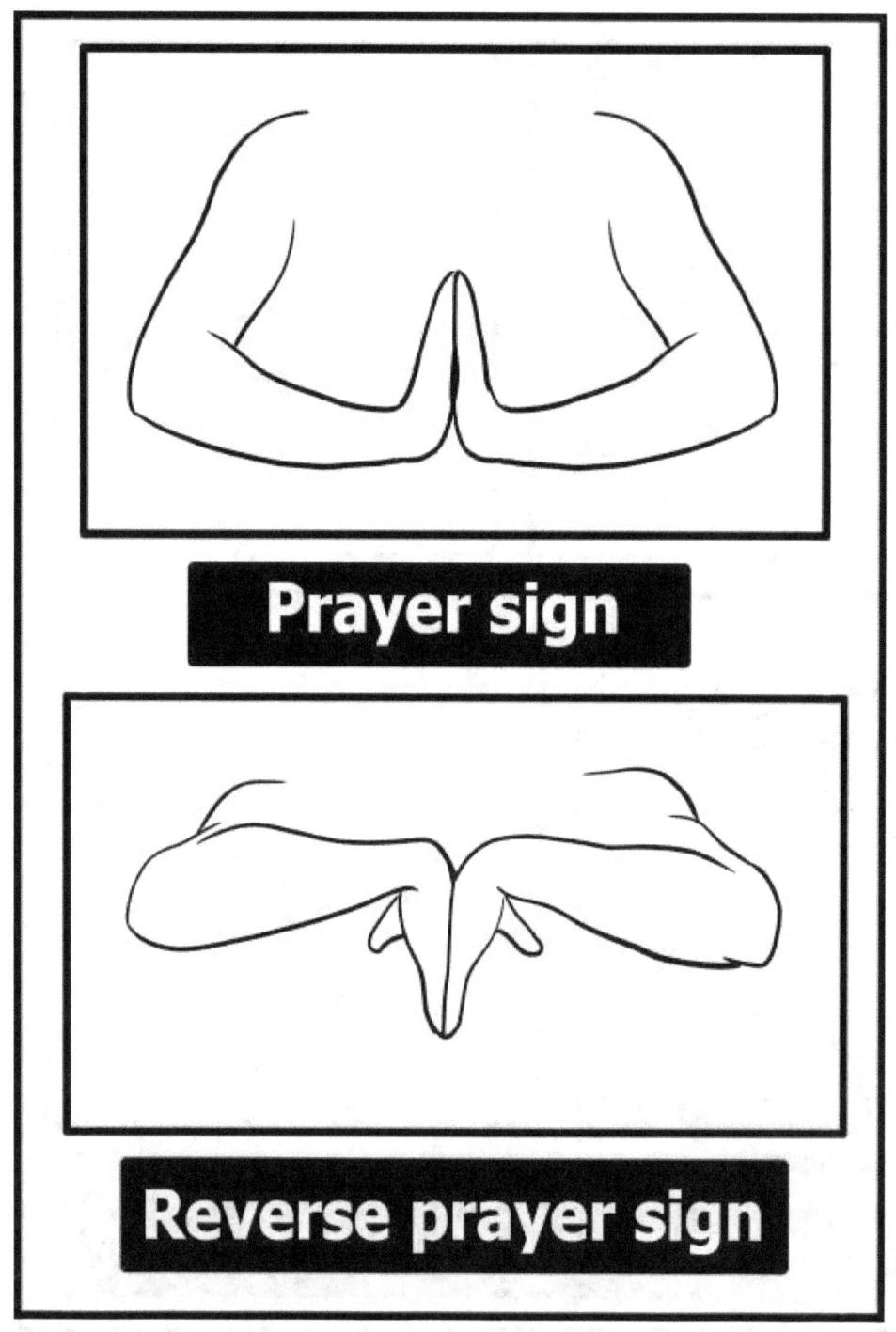

## Hand Examination

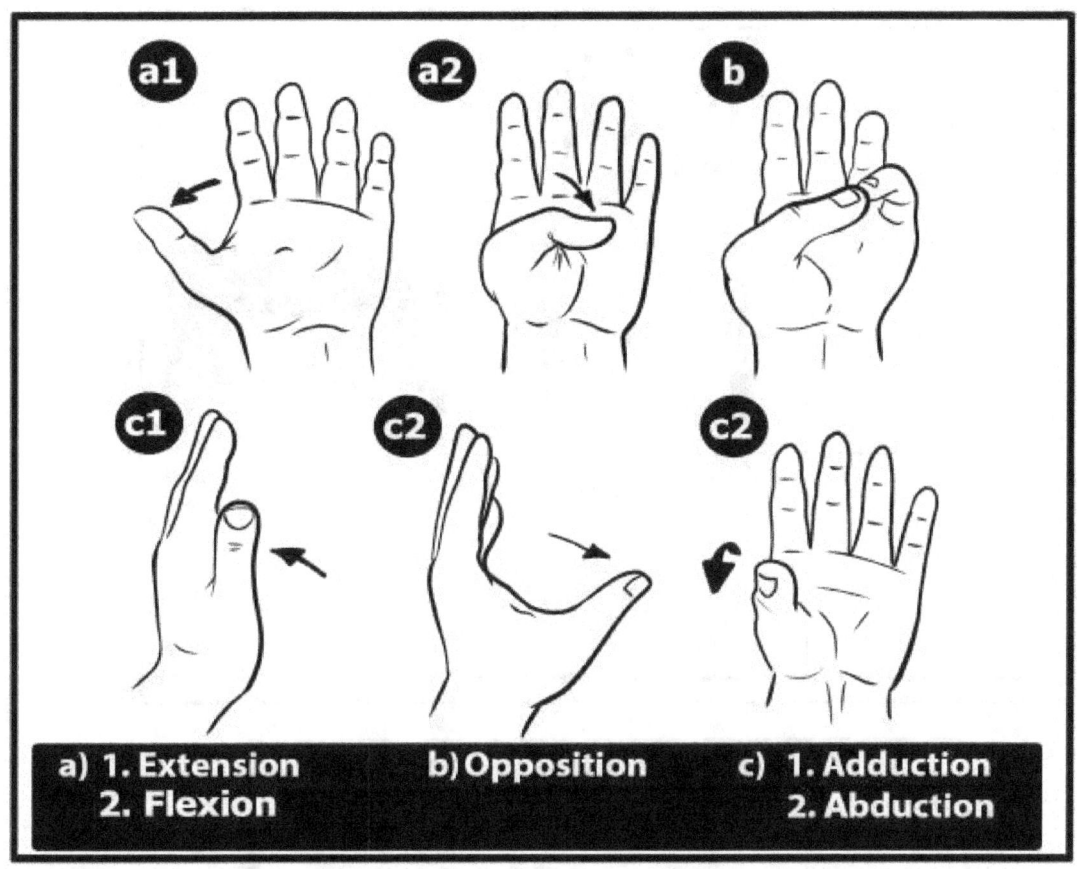

a) 1. Extension  2. Flexion
b) Opposition
c) 1. Adduction  2. Abduction

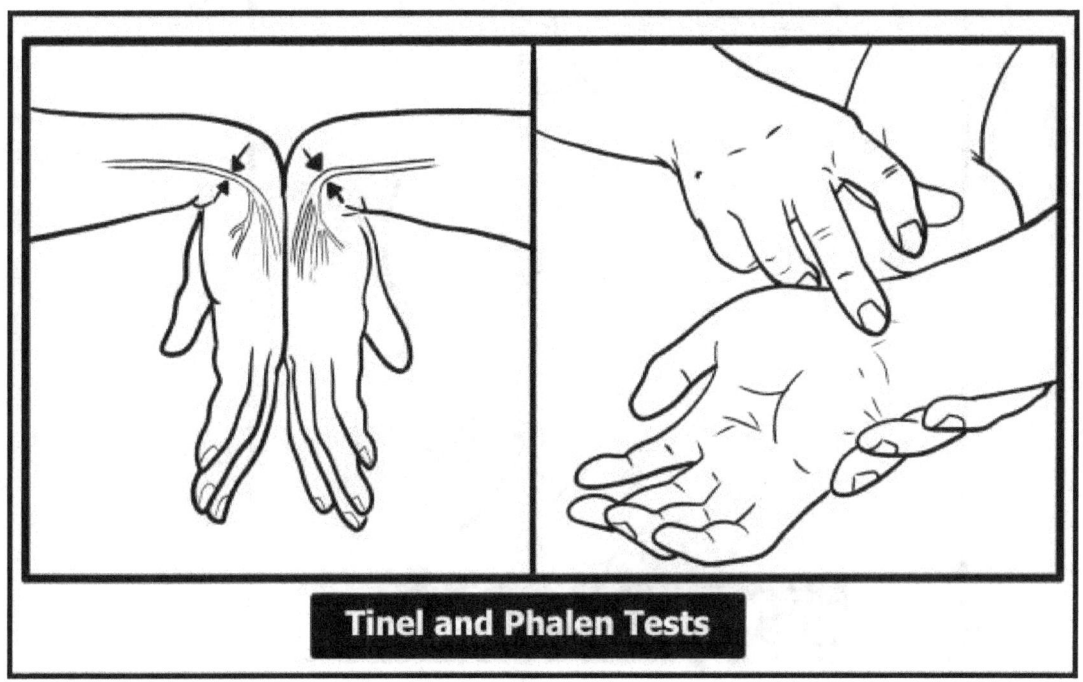

**Tinel and Phalen Tests**

121

# Hand Examination

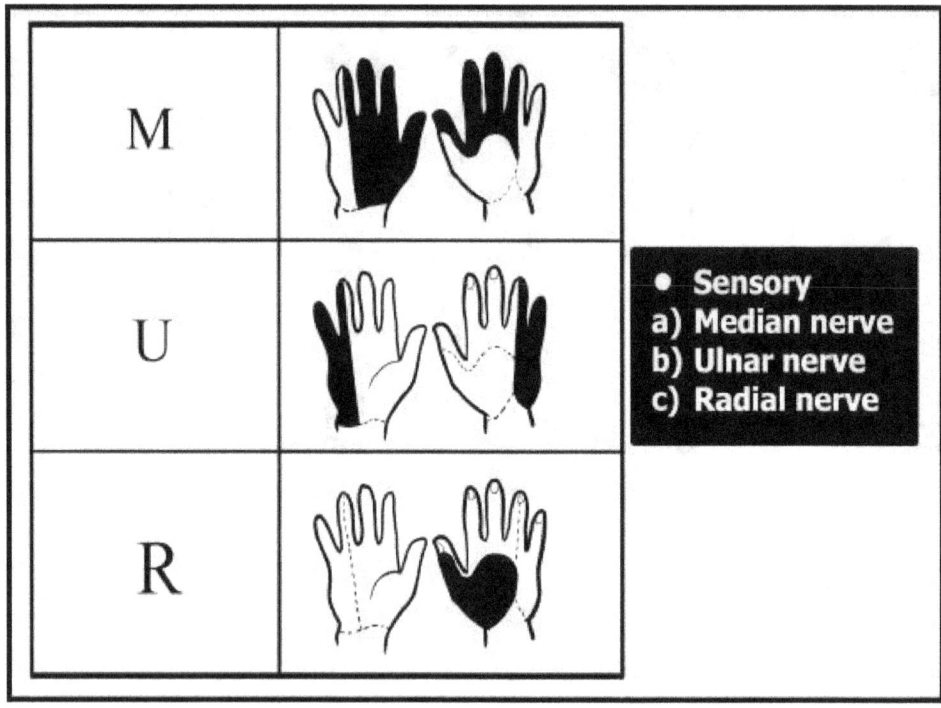

- Sensory
  a) Median nerve
  b) Ulnar nerve
  c) Radial nerve

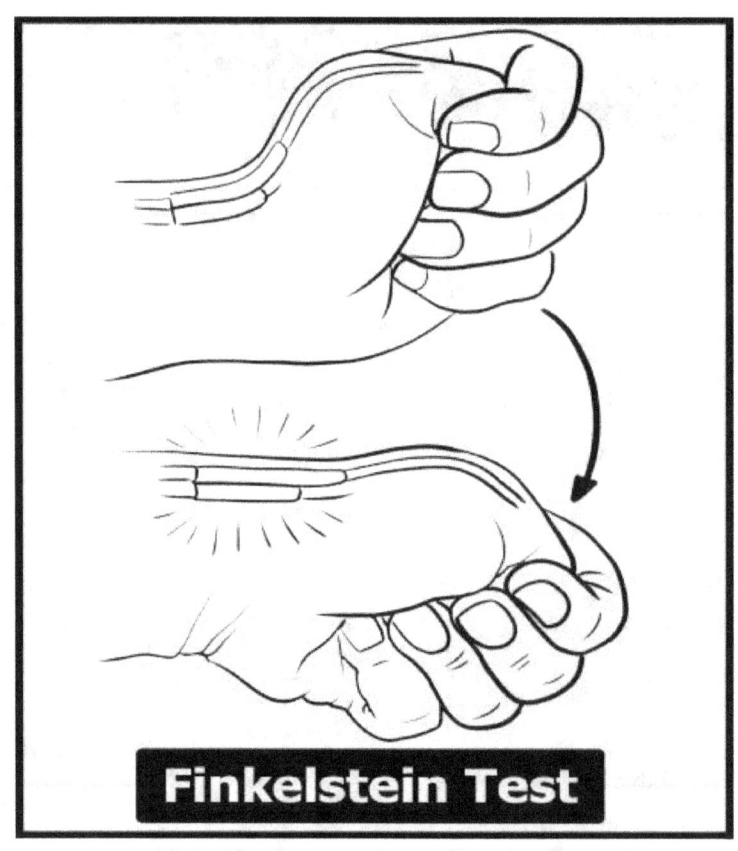

**Finkelstein Test**

# Hand Examination

Dupuytren's contracture

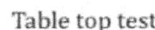
Table top test

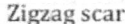
Zigzag scar

## Froment's sign test

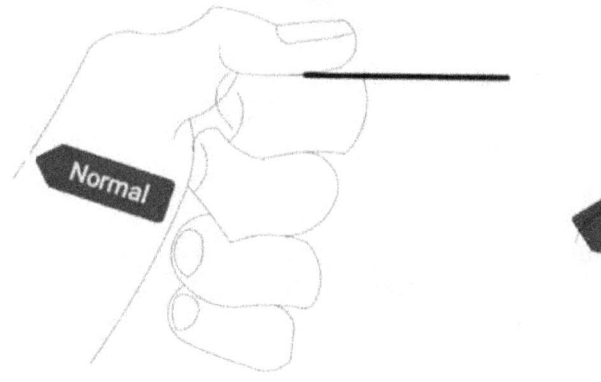

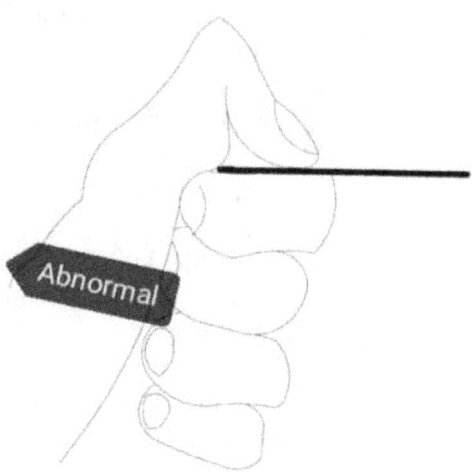

# Hip Examination

| | |
|---|---|
| **General**<br><br>Examine the affected hip or both | 1. Wash hands, introduce yourself, get name and age, explain your roles and gain permission<br>2. Legs exposed wearing only short, supine and one pillow supporting the head<br>3. Around bed (Walking aids, steroid)<br>* steroid causes avascular necrosis. |
| **Inspection** | • **SSSS RAB**<br>- **S**ymmetry<br>- **S**welling (inflammation)<br>- **S**cars (total hip replacement, arthroscopy)<br>- **S**horten leg with externally rotated foot (NOF fractures)<br>- **R**edness (inflammation)<br>- **A**trophy<br>- **B**ruises (trauma)<br>- lumbar lordosis (gap between spine and bed)<br>* Fixed Flexion Deformity(gap between popliteal fossa and bed) is compensated by lumbar lordosis<br><br>• **Pelvic tilt: look at ASIS**<br>* fixed adduction deformity; the ASIS of the deformed side at a higher level and the affected limb appears shortened<br>* fixed abduction deformity; the ASIS of the deformed side at lower level, the affected limb appears lengthened<br>• **Leg length measurement**<br>  1. from umbilicus to medial malleolus: apparent Length<br>  2. from ASIS to medial malleolus: true length<br>• **True limb shortening:**<br>- **Hip:** NOF fracture total hip replacement++dislocation+OA+SUFE +septic arthritis + perthe disease<br>- Old tibial fracture, polio<br>• **Apparent limb shortening:** fixed adduction, flexion, abduction deformity |
| **Palpation** | • Temperature with back of hands over greater trochanter, hip joint<br>• **Tenderness:**<br>a. Joint (deep hardly to find)<br>b. ASIS, greater trochanter (trochanteric bursitis).<br>c. femoral artery: reduced pulsation in dislocated hip (Vascular sign of Narath) |

# Hip Examination

| | |
|---|---|
| **Movement** | - **ROM**<br>  - active vs passive (stabilize the opposite pelvis during abduction and adduction)\\<br><br>  1. **Flexion (120°):** iliopsoas<br>  2. **Extension (10°):** gluteus maximus<br>  3. **Abductor (45°):** gluteus medius and minimus.<br>  4. **Adductor (30°):** abductor group<br>  5. **External rotation (40°):** Internal and external obturators, quadratus femoris superior and inferior gemelli<br>  6. **Internal rotation (40°):** iliopsoas<br><br>- **Decreased ROM in OA** (especially internal rotation) |
| **Palpation** | - Temperature with back of hands over greater trochanter, hip joint<br><br>- **Tenderness:**<br>  a. Joint (deep hardly to find)<br>  b. ASIS, greater trochanter (trochanteric bursitis).<br>  c. femoral artery: reduced pulsation in dislocated hip (Vascular sign of Narath) |
| **Special tests** | 1. **Thomas's test:**<br>   - Fixed flexion deformity(OA) is compensated by lumbar lordosis<br>   - patient supine with extended legs<br>   - feel for any gap (lumbar lordosis) by placing your hand between lumbar spine and bed<br>   - ask patient to bring one knee as far to the chest<br>   - fully flex the hip with one hand while the other beneath patient to assure lumbar spine flatten<br>   - positive sign: if contralateral hip is lifted off the table<br><br>2. **Trendelenburg test:**<br>   - Hip abductor muscle(gluteus medius and gluteus minimum) is supplied superior gluteal nerve |

## Hip Examination

| | |
|---|---|
| | - **Causes:**<br>  - Hip dislocation, osteoarthritis, leg length discrepancy, or abductor weakness, hip dysplasia,<br>  • patient standing in front of you while you're sitting in a chair<br>  • place your hands on iliac crests<br>  • Ask patient to raise one leg<br>  • Iliac crest of the lifted leg will raise which means the contralateral gluteus medius and gluteus minimus are healthy<br>  • If iliac crest of the lifted leg dropped then positive test and the contralateral muscle are weak |
| **Standing** | • Look at Spine (fixed abduction and adduction deformity compensated by scoliosis)<br>• Gluteal atrophy(OA)<br>• **Assess gait:**<br>a. Waddling gait<br>b. Antalgic gait (reduced stance phase on the affected hip) |
| **The End** | • Joint above and below (spine, knee)<br>• Neurovascular examination |

❖ **Hip fractures: Intracapsular VS Extracapsular**

- **Complication:**
  Nonunion, avascular necrosis, thromboembolism(fat embolism),bed sore

A. **Intracapsular(above to intertrochanteric line)**
1. **Neck of femur :**

- **Risk factors :**
- Elderly (osteoporosis),falls into sides(into greater trochanter)

- **Clinical features:**
- Pain (hip, groin)
- ROM restricted
- Unable to carry weight
- Leg is abducted , externally rotated and shorten

## Hip Examination

- **Classification:**
- Garden:
- **Type 1:(Nondisplaced)** incomplete fracture
- **Type 2:(Nondisplaced)** complete fracture
- **Type 3:(Displaced)** complete with partial displaced
- **Type 4:(Displaced)** complete and fully displaced

- **XRAY:**
- Abnormal shenton line

- **Treatment:**
- **ORIF: young Pt with displaced fracture**
- cannulated screw fixation: Nondisplaced
- Total hip replacement (THR) or Hemiarthroplasty:
- Elderly Pt with displaced
- Preexisting severe degenerative joint

- **Indications THR:**
- Severe RA, OA
- Osteoporosis
- Disabling

2. **Extracapsular (at intertrochanteric line and below it)**

    **Intertrochanteric (at intertrochanteric line) & subtrochanteric (below the line) fracture**
    - Internal fixation and dynamic hip screw

❖ **Hip dislocation :**

- **Posterior hip dislocation:** Sciatic nerve palsy
- **Anterior hip dislocation (rare):** Femoral nerve injury

## Hip Examination

### 1. Osteoarthritis:
- Joints involved commonly (knee ,hip ,DIP ,PIP ,spine)

- **Risk factors:**
- Female ,Age ,obesity
- Trauma
- Gout ,Rheumatoid arthritis
- Childhood diseases (Perthes disease, DDH)

- **Clinical features:**
- Chronic Stiffness/pain
- Decreased ROM
- Worsen with activity (at end of day)&improve with rest
- Antalgic or Trendelenburg gait.
- Flexion and adduction deformity
- Varus flexion knee
- Tenderness on joint line palpation
- Crepitus with movement(knee noise)

- **X RAY:**
  - **L** – loss of joint space
  - **O** – osteophytes
  - **S** – subchondral sclerosis
  - **S** – subchondral cyst

- **Treatment**
  - Weight loss
  - Paracetamol
  - NSAIDs:
- **Side effects**: (gastric: ulceration, perforation, hemorrhage)
  - If high risk of bleeding supplement with omeprazole (PPI) avoid in PUD/CRF
  - Triamcinolone (Intra-articular injections for hip and knee )
  - Total hip replacement
  - Indications for pain at rest or restricted movement ,dysfunction, failure of medication

- **DD of hip pain:**
  - Lumbar radiculopathy
  - Strain
  - Bursitis
  - OA
  - RA
  - Septic arthritis

### 2. Osteoporosis:

## Hip Examination

- low bone mass

- **Risk factors:**
- Age , female , postmenopausal state , low BMI , steroid, multiple myeloma , hyperthyroidism.
- **Present as :**
- spinal kyphosis
- colles fracture
- hip fracture

- **Investigation:**
- Dexa Scan:
- T-score
a. -1.0 and -2.5 (osteopenia)
b. -2.5 and below (osteoporosis)

- **Treatment :**
- Bisphosphonates
- Calcitonin
- Estrogen
- denosumab

# Hip Examination

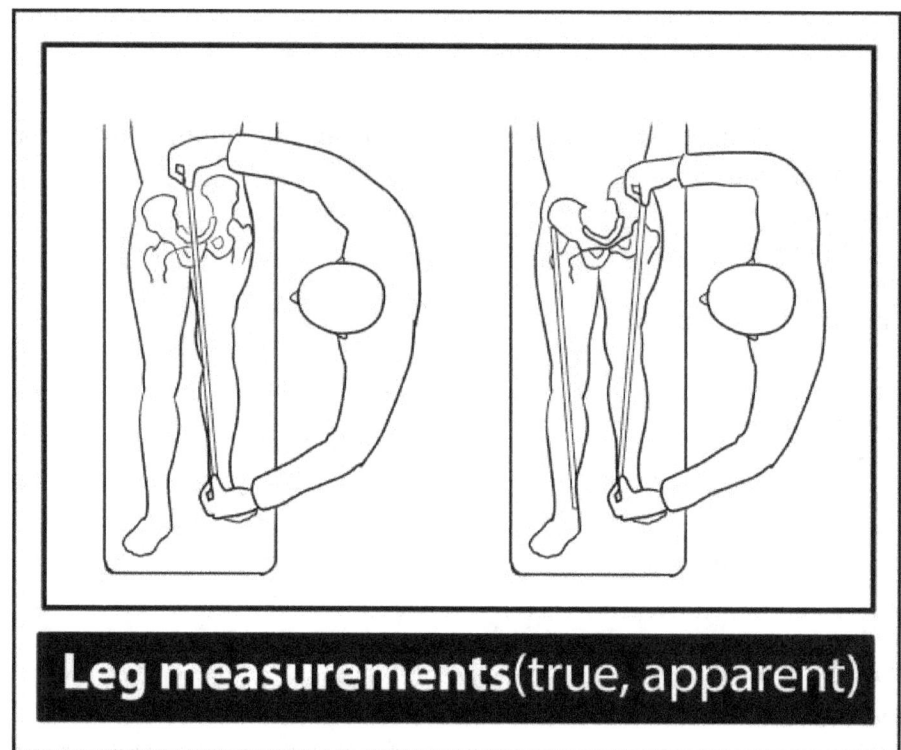

**Leg measurements** (true, apparent)

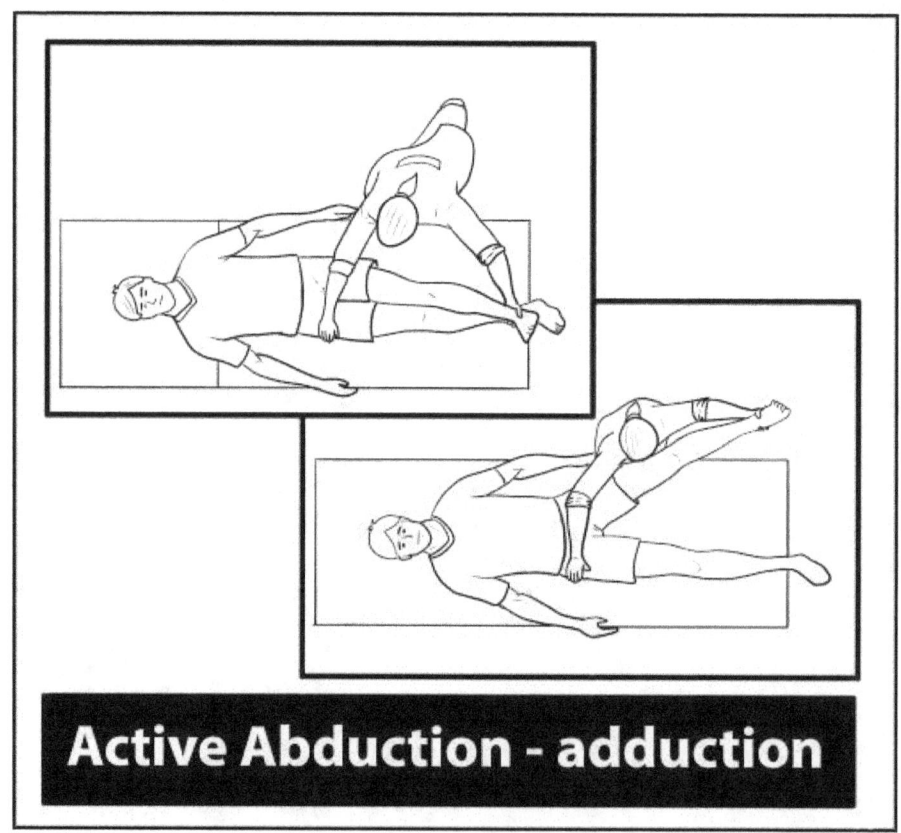

**Active Abduction - adduction**

## Hip Examination

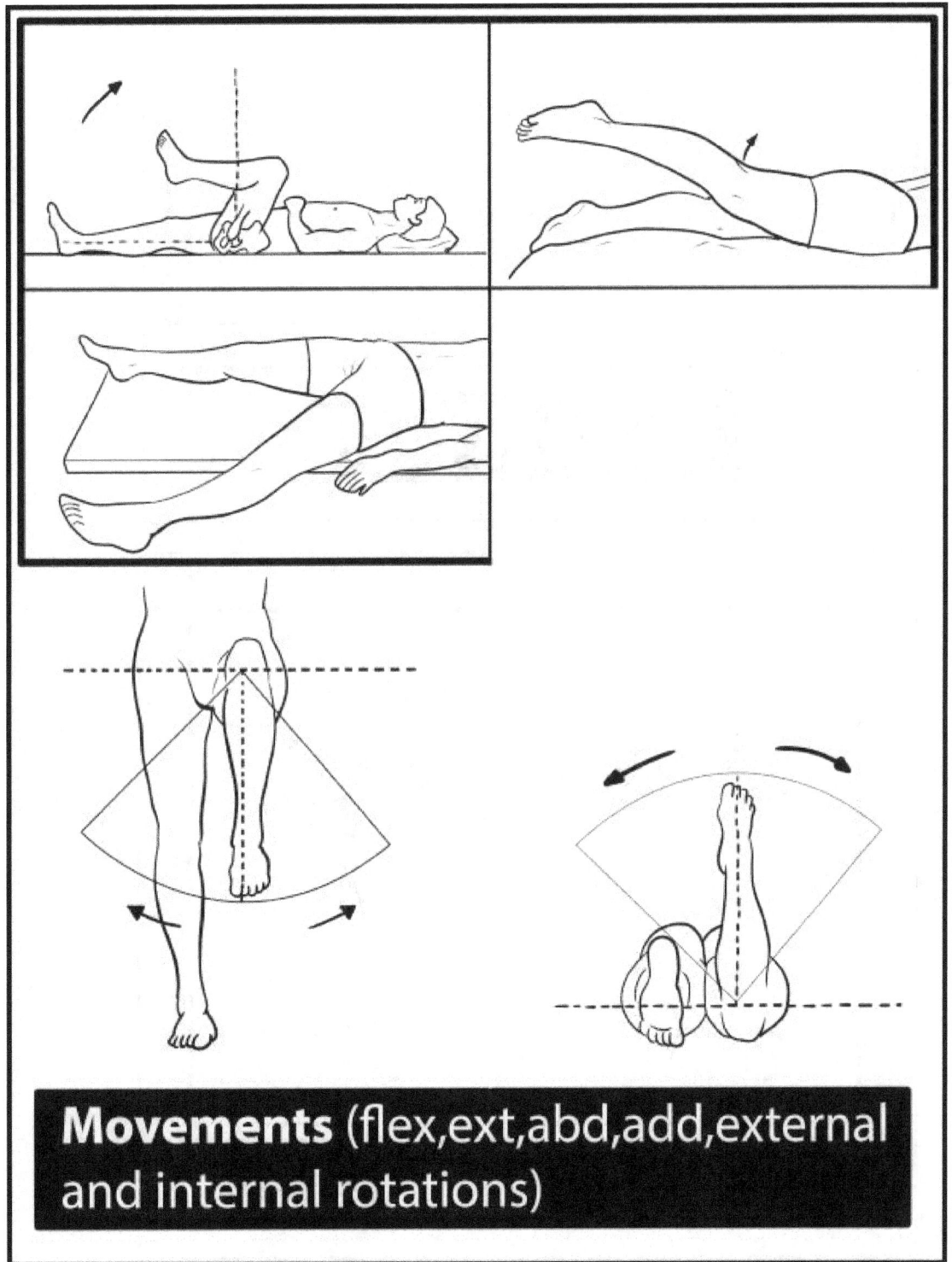

**Movements** (flex, ext, abd, add, external and internal rotations)

## Hip Examination

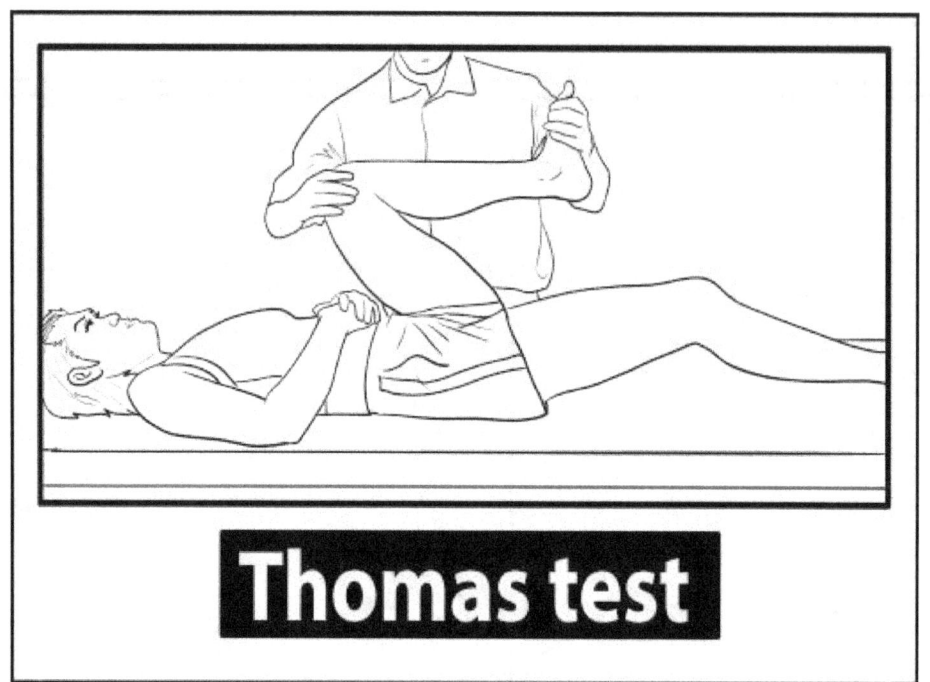

**Thomas test**

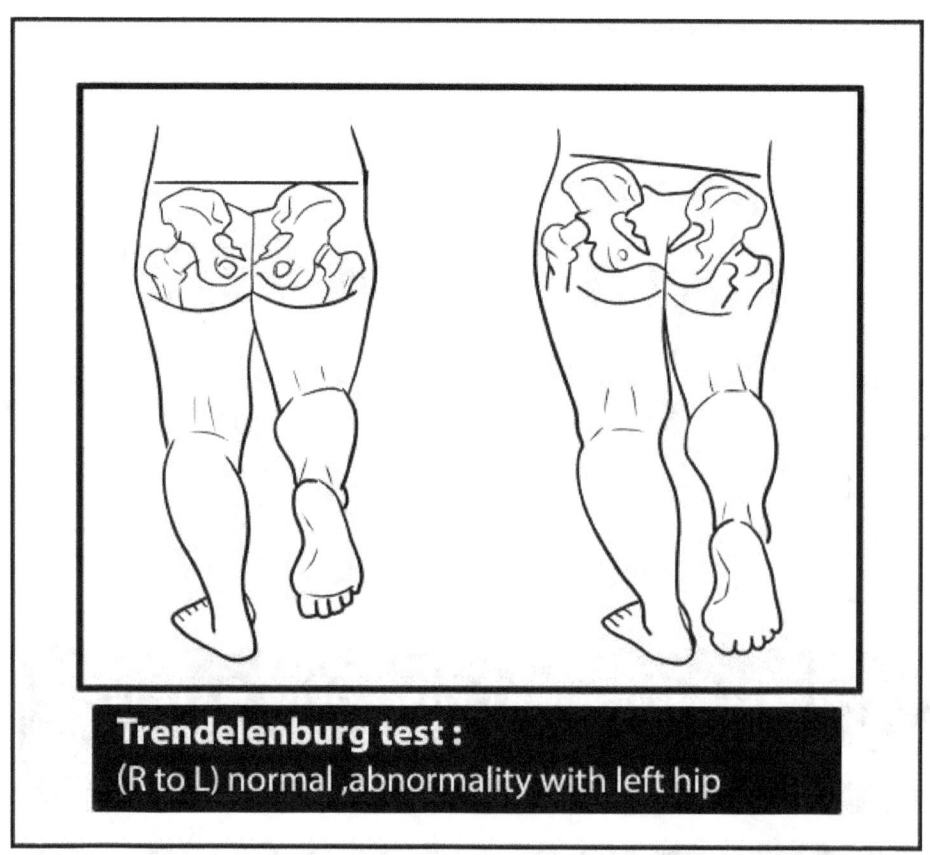

**Trendelenburg test:**
(R to L) normal, abnormality with left hip

# Knee Examination

| | |
|---|---|
| **General**<br><br>Examine the affected knee or both | 1. Wash hands, introduce yourself, get name and age, explain your roles and gain permission<br>2. Legs exposed wearing only short, lying at 45 degrees bed<br>3. Around bed (Walking aids,) |
| **Inspection** | ▪ **Compare both sides**<br>❖ **Patient standing:**<br>1. Assess gait<br>- antalgic gait (reduced stance phase on the affected hip)<br>2. Scars: arthroscopy(meniscectomy), midline longitudinal incisions (knee replacement)<br>3. Swelling, erythema(inflammation)<br>4. Plaque psoriasis<br>5. Wasting (Quadriceps): measure 15 cm above superior pole of patella<br>6. Baker cyst in popliteal area (RA, OA) treated by synovectomy<br>7. Deformities:(increases the risk of OA)<br>a) Flexion deformity (knee locked unable to extend)<br>b) Varus (OA)and valgus deformity (arthritis) |
| **Palpation** | 1. Temperature use back of hand above knee (inflammation, Septic arthritis)<br>2. Tenderness:<br>• Knee must be flexed at 90 degrees, ask if it causing any pain<br>• Popliteal areal (baker cyst)<br>• Medial and lateral side (collateral ligaments, meniscus injury)<br>• Patella borders<br>• Tibial tuberosity (Tibial apophysitis)<br>• Femoral condyles<br><br>1. **Effusion Tests:**<br>- **On Lying position**<br>a) **Patellar tap (large effusion):**<br>• Slide your hand down on thigh<br>• Compress firmly above suprapatellar pouch<br>• Using index and middle finger of the other hand to press patella down<br>• **positive**= patellae bounces off |

# Knee Examination

| | |
|---|---|
| | **b) Bulge sign (small fluid):**<br>• Swipe your hand upward in the medial aspect of knee few time then hold up your hand in top<br>• Using your other hand swipe downward the lateral aspect<br>• Positive = appearance of bulge in the medial side |
| **Movement** | ▪ **ROM**<br>• Active VS passive (hands placed over knee feeling for crepitus)<br>• Flexion 140(biceps femoris + semitendinosus)<br>• Extension (quadriceps femoris)<br>• Hyperextension (10 degrees) |
| **Special Tests**<br><br>**Patient lying flat** | 1. **Anterior drawer test (ACL tear), Posterior drawer test(PCL)**<br>• Knee flexed at 90 degrees<br>• Sit on the foot<br>• Hold the upper tibia with both hands (fingers behind the knee, thumbs on patella)<br>• Pull the leg toward yourself(anteriorly) for ACL<br>• Push away from you (posteriorly)<br>• Compare both knees for anterior or posterior translations (displacement) of the tibia<br><br>2. **Lachman's test(ACL)**<br>• One hand stabilize the femur(above the knee)<br>• The other hand pull tibia anteriorly and posteriorly<br>• Assess for laxity<br><br>3. **Collateral ligament test (medial and lateral)**<br>• One hand holding the calf off the bed and stabilizing the leg (knee flexed at 30 degree)<br>• One hand in lateral aspect of the knee applying stress in inward direction(MCL)<br>• one hand in the medial aspect of the knee applying stress in outward direction(LCL)<br>• Positive if any abnormal excessive movement in medial or lateral direction |

# Knee Examination

4. **McMurray's test**
Positive = pain /click

- Both hip and knee flexed at 90 degrees

A. **Lateral meniscal injury**
- one hand over lateral joint line of knee
- the other hand holding the heel and internally rotate the foot (big toe is inward) and extend it, redo it again at different angles while varus(bring knee outward) force is applied

B. **medial meniscal injury**
- One hand over medial joint line of knee
- The other hand holding the heel and externally rotate the foot (foot is outward) then extend it, redo it again at different angles while valgus force applied(bring knee inward )

5. **Patellar apprehension test:**
- With both thumbs apply lateral force in the medial aspect of patella
- **positive= pain (patellar dislocation, patellofemoral syndrome)**
- **Other**: Apply grind test for meniscal injury

**The End**
- Offer to examine the joint above and the joint below neurological and vascular examination of the limb examined

## 1. Gout:

- **Seen in :**
- Obesity, male, Beer binging, leukemia, thiazide

- **Clinical features:**
- **Acute** : Monoarthritis (1 MTP, lower limb joints), warm, erythema, tender, fever
- **Chronic** : recurrent acute attacks or Tophus(ear) **specific**, Uric Acid stone

- **Investigations:**
- **Blood**: Hyperuricemia, WCC
- **Arthrocentesis**: uric acid crystal (needle-shaped, negatively birefringent), high WCC
- **Radiology**: punched-out lesion, rat bite erosion

# Knee Examination

- **Treatment:**
- **Lifestyle modification**: weight loss, avoid Dietary purine and alcohol,
  - **Acute:**
    - NSAID
    - Colchicine
    - Steroid
  - **Long term:**
    - **Uric lowering:**
    a. Xanthine oxidase inhibitors (allopurinol)
    - **Side effects**: Hypersensitivity pruritic rash especially in HLA-B*5801 so screening
    b. Uricosuric agents (probenecid)
    c. Uricase (pegloticase)

## 2. PseudoGout:

- **Risk factors**: HHH
  - Hyperparathyroidism
  - Hemochromatosis
  - Hypothyroidism

- **Clinical features:**
  - Monoarthritis (knee), warm, erythema
  - Elderly

- **Investigations:**
  - **Arthrocentesis**: calcium pyrophosphate crystals (rhomboid shape, positively birefringent)
  - **Radiology**: chondrocalcinosis

- **Treatment:**
  - NSAID
  - Colchicine
  - Intra-articular steroid

## 3. Septic arthritis:
- **S. aureus**

- **Risk factors:**
  - Injections
  - Surgery
  - artificial joint
  - Immunosuppression

- **Clinical features:**

# Knee Examination

- Fever
- Acute monoarthritis, tender, erythema, swelling(knee)

- **Investigations**
- **Synovial fluid aspiration:** PMN, WBC, Gram stain, purulent colour
- **blood**: WCC, CRP

- **Treatment**
- Joint fluid drainage +IV antibiotic

❖ **Knee pathologies:**

1. **Ligaments:**

a. **ACL**:
- **injuries:**
  - Hyperextension of knee
  - Fall on twisted knee then hearing audible pop sound followed by immediate early effusion and , hemarthrosis)
  - Painful unstable knee
* **Unhappy triad**: ACL, MCL, medial meniscus injuries

b. **PCL**:
- Injuries:
  - Hyperflexion of knee(PCL)
  - dashboard injury

c. **collateral ligaments**
- medial >lateral
- **injuries**: Trauma on the lateral or medial sides of knee
- painful knee with little effusion

2. **Meniscal tears:**
- **Risk factors:** Discoid meniscus
- Injuries
  - Young male who twist his weight-bearing knee while flexed
  - Painful knee followed hours later by effusion
  - Locked knee (inability to extend to knee)
  - Wasting of the quadriceps
  - Joint line tenderness
  - **DD of hip pain:** fractures, dislocation, rupture of the quadriceps tendon, Iliotibial band syndrome, patellofemoral syndrome

# Knee Examination

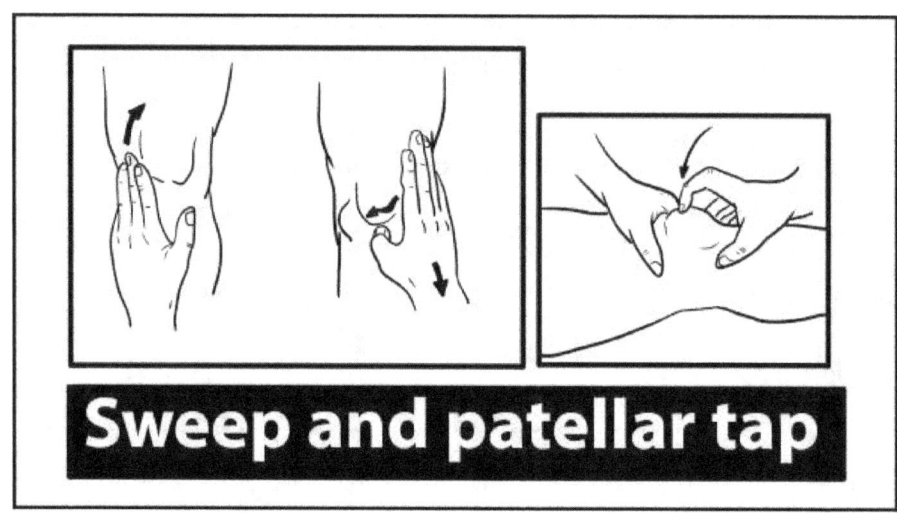

Sweep and patellar tap

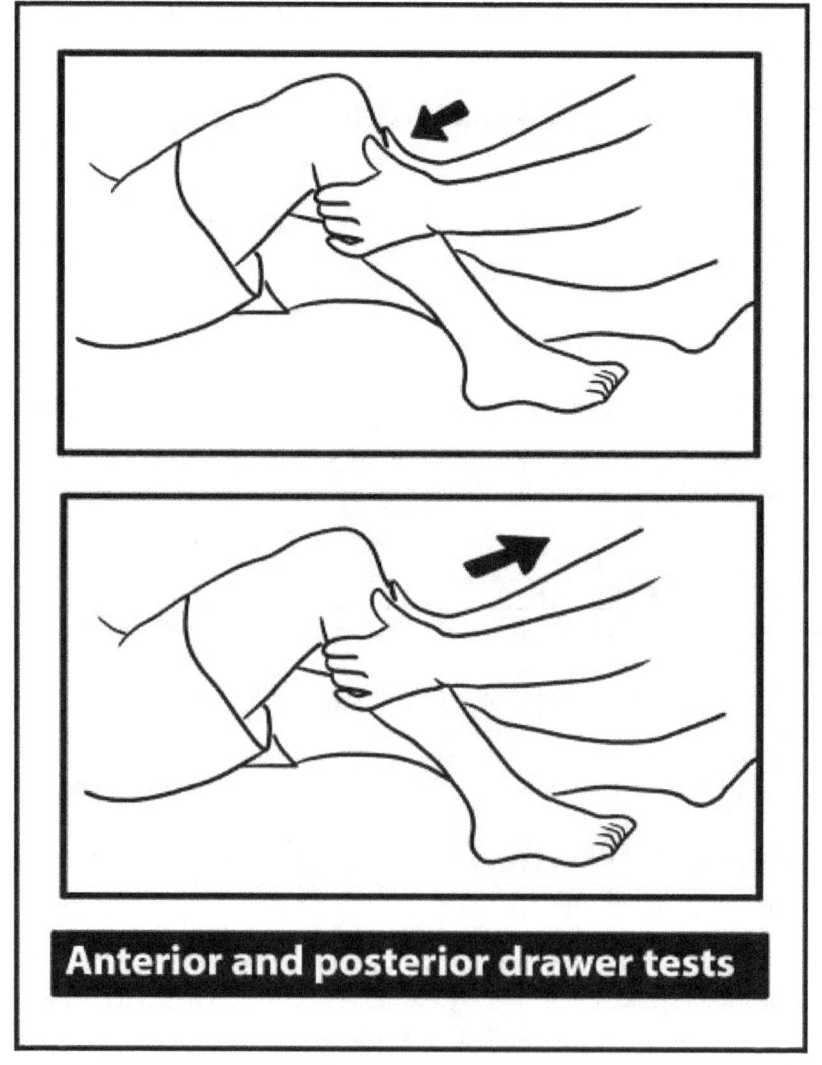

Anterior and posterior drawer tests

## Knee Examination

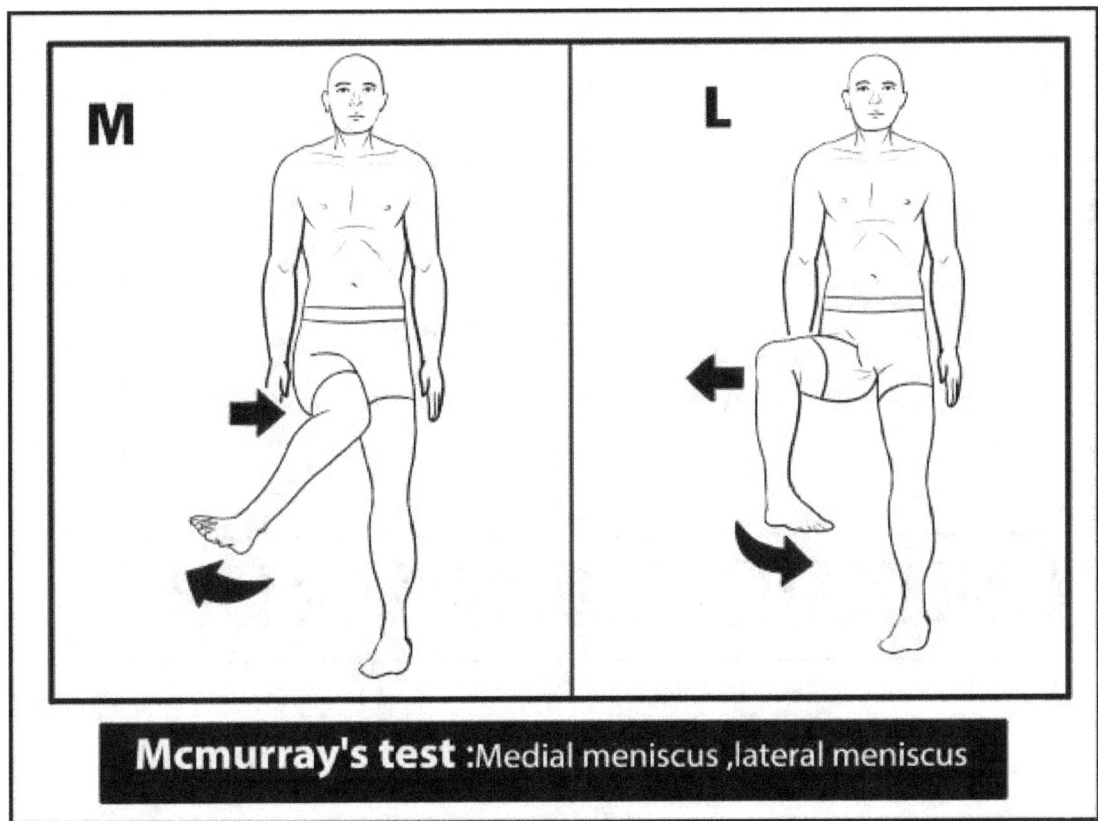

**Mcmurray's test**: Medial meniscus, lateral meniscus

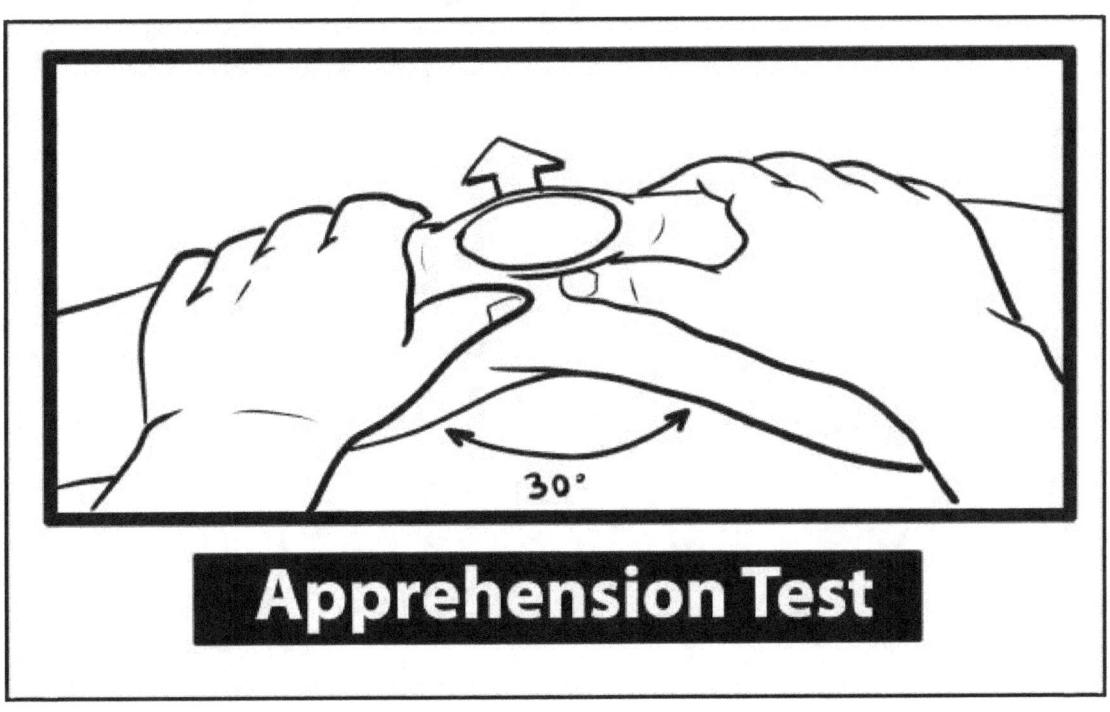

**Apprehension Test**

## Knee Examination

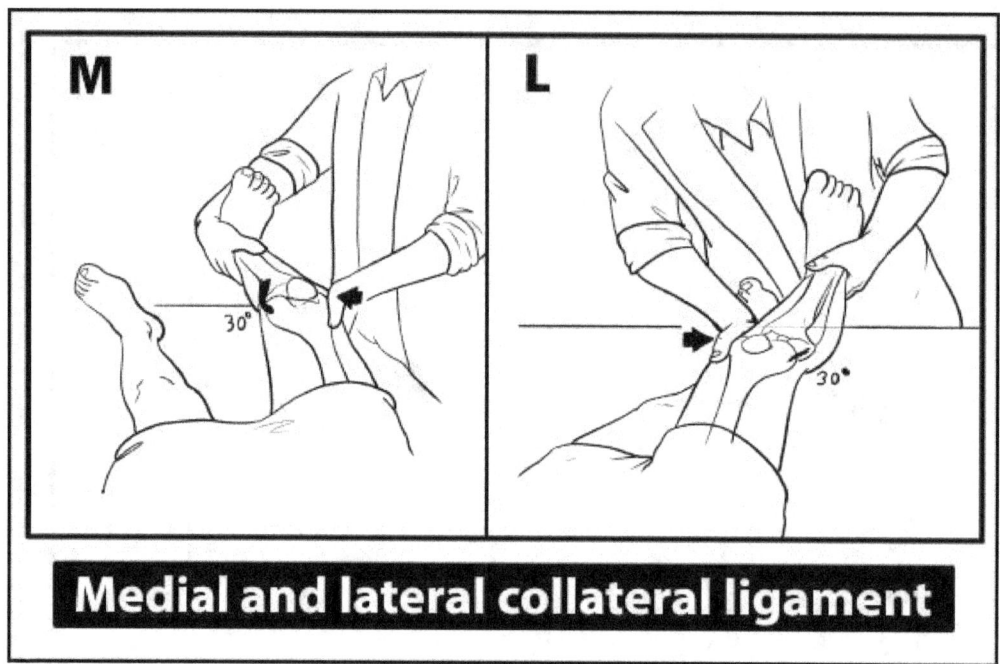

**Medial and lateral collateral ligament**

# Spine Examination

| | |
|---|---|
| **General** | 1. Wash your hands<br>2. Introduce yourself<br>3. Gain permission<br>4. PT must be standing up and wearing short |
| **Look** | • Front, sides and back<br>• For normal cervical lordosis, thoracic kyphosis and lumbar lordosis<br>• For scoliosis (Ankylosing Spondylitis)<br>• Question mark posture:<br>- loss of lumbar lordosis<br>- thoracic kyphosis<br>- Cervical hyperextension<br>- Pot belly |
| **Feel (tenderness, temperature)** | - Palpate with tips of your fingers each spinal vertebra & sacroiliac joints<br>- Palpate both sides of spine (paravertebral muscles) with both of your hands at the same time |
| **Move** | ▪ **Active only.**<br>• **Actively:**<br>1. Lumbar<br>  a. flexion (touch your toes)<br>  b. extension (lean backwards)<br>  c. lateral flexion (run your hand down on outside of your leg to the left and right)<br>2. Cervical:<br>- Touch ear to shoulder (lateral flexion)<br>- Look up (extension)<br>- Look down (flexion)<br>- Look left (rotation)<br>- Look right (rotation)<br><br>• **Thoracic rotation:**<br>- Ask patient to sit on the edge of bed with his arms crossed<br>- Fix his pelvis with your hands<br>- Ask PT Rotate to left and right |

## Spine Examination

| | |
|---|---|
| **Special tests:** | • **Stretch test or straight leg raise:**<br>- Actively flex PT hip while his knee is extended<br>- Positive if pain on posterior leg is elicited between 30-70 degrees (lumbar disc herniation at L4-S1)<br><br>• **Femoral nerve stretch test:**<br>- Actively extend PT hip while PT on prone position with fixed knee.<br>- Positive if pain on anterior leg (impingement at L2,3,4)<br><br>• **Schobert's test (lumbar flexion)**<br>- While patient is standing<br>- Find level L5 at PSIS (dimple) and make imaginary line.<br>- Mark two points 5 cm below and 10 cm above this line<br>- Ask patient to touch his toes while his knees straight.<br>- Premeasure the distance between the two points if the distance of the two points not increased by 5cms or not 20 cms in total then the test is positive (ankylosing spondylitis)<br>- The occiput to wall distance tests (thoracic kyphosis)<br>- Ask the PT to lay his back against a wall<br>- Positive if PT is unable to place his occiput on wall |
| **The End** | • **Offer to do:**<br>- Offer to examine the joint above and the joint below<br>- AS complications:<br>Lung (apical fibrosis)<br>Chest expansion (reduced)<br>Heart (aortic incompetence)<br>-<br>neurological examination<br>- X-ray or MRI of spine |

- **Complication of AS**
- Anterior uveitis
- Restrictive lung disease and pulmonary fibrosis
- Aortic valve insufficiency, AV blocks
- Osteoporosis
- Cauda equina syndrome

## Upper Limb Neurological Examination

| | |
|---|---|
| **General** | 1. Wash hands, introduce yourself, get name and age, explain your role out pain and gain permission<br>2. At 45 degrees, arms exposed or shirt off<br>3. Always compare both arms<br>4. Ask Pt to put the back of his hands on his thighs<br>5. Around bed: drugs, Mobility Aids<br>6. Patient: posture, speech, hemispatial neglect syndrome |
| **Inspection** | • Wasting:<br>- Flattened deltoid (axillary N palsy due to fractured surgical neck of humerus or anterior dislocation of humerus)<br>- Dorsal interosseous +thenar (median N palsy)<br>- Hypothenar (ulnar N palsy)<br>• Asymmetry, deformity<br>• Scars<br>• Fasciculation (deltoid, biceps): if it is not clear tap with hammer to elicit<br>• Abnormal Position<br>• Deformity : erb's palsy, klumpke.<br>• Upper limb flexion(decorticate), upper limb extension (decerebrate) in stroke<br>• Involuntary movement:<br>a. Asymmetrical rest tremor (parkinson)<br>b. Postural (against gravity with spread fingers) and action:<br>1. Essential tremor (symmetrical upper limb, head tremors improved with alcohol)<br>2. Physiological tremor (coffee, stress, hyperthyroidism, Beta agonist)<br>c. Intention tremor (cerebellar, MS)<br><br>*postural tremor is worse when patient arms outstretched and spread fingers<br><br>• Pronator drift test (dorsal column UMN lesion)<br>- Eyes closed with both arm outstretched and palms facing the roof (supinated)<br>- Positive if one of hand pronated(palmar side of hand faces floor) |
| **Tone** | • Hypertonia (UMN lesion or parkinson):<br>- Spasticity<br>- Rigidity<br>• Hypotonia (LMN lesion, cerebellar disease)<br>- Shoulder: abduction, adduction<br>- Elbow: flexion, extension<br>- Wrist: flexion, extension, supination, pronation |

## Upper Limb Neurological Examination

| | |
|---|---|
| **Power** | - **Grade power in these moments with muscle isolation(support above joint):**<br>- **Compare**<br>  - Shoulder: abduction<br>  - Elbow: flexion, extension<br>  - Wrist: extension<br>  - Fingers: flexion, extension, abduction(bring your index away from the fingers and hold the other three fingers in your hand and try push the index back to them)<br>  - Thumb: abduction(bring your thumb toward yourself)<br><br>- **MRC grade 0-5:**<br>0. no movement<br>1. flicker of movement<br>2. movement with gravity eliminated (Pt is not able to abduct his arm but when he lay supine on bed, he can abduct his arm )<br>3. movement against gravity(Pt able to abduct his shoulder but can't resist you and his hands will go down quickly)<br>4. movement against resistance, not full strength<br>5. normal power for age and sex |
| **Reflexes** | \* **maneuver to reinforce reflexes:** clench teeth<br>Look at the muscle not the reflex<br><br>- **Biceps**: C5/C6<br>- **Triceps**: C7<br>- **brachioradialis**: C5/C6<br><br>- **0** absent<br>- **1** diminished seen with reinforcement<br>- **2** Normal<br>- **3** Hyperactive without clonus<br>- **4** Hyperactive with clonus |
| **Coordination** | - **Cerebellar lesion**<br>  - Finger-nose test<br>  - Past pointing(dysmetria), intention tremor<br>  - Rapid alternating movements(Dysdiadochokinesia) |

# Upper Limb Neurological Examination

| Sensation | <ul><li>**Test on sternum, eyes closed**</li><li>**Light touch and pin-prick**</li></ul>  - **C4** shoulder  - **C5** medial arm (badges)  - **C6** thumb  - **C7** middle finger  - **C8** little finger  - **T1** medial part middle of forearm  <ul><li>**Proprioception**:</li></ul>  - holding the medial and lateral sides of ines and move the distal phalanx up and down  - If not felt move to wrist , elbow  <ul><li>**Vibration** (128 Hz)</li></ul>  - Index tip  - If not felt move to radial styloid, ocleron |
|---|---|
| **The End** | <ul><li>Hoffmann's reflex for UMN Lesions above T1</li><li>Examine lower limb nerves and cranial nerves</li></ul> |

|  | **Movement (Muscle)** | **Nerve** |
|---|---|---|
| **Shoulder** | Abduction(Deltoid) | Axillary C5 |
| **Elbow** | Flexion(Biceps) | Musculocutaneous(C5,6) |
| **Elbow** | Extension (Triceps) | Radial C7 |
| **Wrist** | Extension (Extensor carpi ulnaris) | Radial (C7) |
| **Fingers** | Extension (extensor digitorum) | Radial (C7) |
| **Fingers** | Flexion (flexor digitorum) | Median +ulnar(C8) |
| **Fingers** | Abduction (Interossei muscle) | Ulnar(T1) |
| **Thumb** | Abduction (Abductor pollicis brevis) | Median (T1) |

## Upper Limb Neurological Examination

| UMN lesion | LMN lesion |
|---|---|
| - Hypertonia<br>- Hyperreflexia<br>- Babinski sign (+)<br>- Atrophy from disuse (later)<br>- Spastic paralysis on:<br>  a. **Contralateral: lesion** above pyramidal decussation<br>  b. **Ipsilateral :** below it | - Hypotonia<br>- Hyporeflexia<br>- Fasciculation<br>- Muscle atrophy<br>- Flaccid paralysis or weakness in the same side of the lesion |
| - Brain pathology is **unilateral** : tumor, abscess, stroke, hemorrhage, MS, TIA<br>- spinal pathology is **bilateral** : spianl stenosis, disc herniation, fracture, MS, | - DM, GBS, vasculitis, chemotherapy |

| Dorsal column pathway (ascending) | Spinothalamic pathway (ascending) | Lateral corticospinal pathway (descending) |
|---|---|---|
| - Pressure<br>- Vibration<br>- Fine touch<br>- Proprioception | - Pain<br>- Temperature | - Voluntary movements |

| Syringomyelia | Brown-Séquard Syndrome |
|---|---|
| - Expansion of syrinx (cervical spine) due to spinal tumor, Arnold-Chiari malformation<br>- Early signs (spinothalamic): bilateral loss of pain and temperature in cape-like distribution mainly upper limb )<br>- Late sign (expand to anterior horn causing LMN lesion signs): flaccid muscle<br>- horner syndrome<br>- hand muscle atrophy<br>- Thoracic kyphoscoliosis may progress to syringobulbia | - Spinal cord is hemisected due to traumatic injury or spinal tumor<br>1. Ipsilateral loss of vibration, proprioception (dorsal column), paralysis (corticospinal) below the level of lesion<br>2. contralateral loss of pain and temperature below level of lesion (spinothalamic) |

## Upper Limb Neurological Examination

❖ **Brachial plexus injury**

| Upper lesion (Erb Duchene) | Lower lesion (Klumpke) |
|---|---|
| <ul><li>C5, C6</li><li>waiter's tip position(arm adducted ,elbow flexed and wrist flexed and pronated) muscle atrophy(arm)</li><li>loss of sense of lateral arm & forearm</li></ul> | <ul><li>C8,T1</li><li>total claw hand(atrophy of intrinsic muscle)unlike claw hand of ulnar nerve palsy (medial fingers only)</li><li>loss of senses of medial arm &forearm</li><li>+/- Horner's syndrome</li></ul> |

| | |
|---|---|
| **UMNL** | Hypertonia, hyperreflexia ,weakness, |
| **LMNL** | Hypotonia, Hyporeflexia ,fasciculation and muscle wasting |
| **Muscle disease** | Wasting, hypotonia in a specific muscle group and normmal reflex |
| **NMJ** | <ul><li>Neuromuscular junction disease</li><li>Generalized weakness, which worsen with repetition, normal tone and reflex</li></ul> |

| | |
|---|---|
| **Parkinson** | Hypertonia , normal reflexes, tremor |
| **Cerebellar** | Hypotonia , normal reflexes, coordination test (positive) |

❖ **Stroke:**

a. **Ischemic (mostly):**
- Thrombosis on atherosclerosis (carotid artery, MCA)
- Embolism:
1. **Cardiac source:** AFIB, MI, IE
2. **Artery: carotid**
- **Others**: artery dissection

*same risk factors of MI

## Upper Limb Neurological Examination

b. **Hemorrhagic:**
- Subarachnoid hemorrhage
- Intracerebral hemorrhage brain

- **Clinical feature:**

According to the location

- **MCA:**
- Contralateral upper limb and face paralysis and sensory loss
- Aphasia, agraphia, (dominant side affected left usually)
- Hemispatial neglect syndrome (non-dominant side)
- contralateral homonymous hemianopia

- **ACA:**
- Contralateral Lower limb paralysis and sensory loss
- Personality changes
- urinary in continence

- **PICA :** (Wallenberg syndrome)
- **CN 10** (hoarseness, dysphagia, loss of gag reflex)
- **CN 8** (vertigo, vomiting)
- **CN 5** (loss pain and temperature ipsilateral side of face)
- Sympathetic tract (ipsilateral horner syndrome)
- **Spinothalamic tract** (**contralateral** pain and temperature)

- **Investigations:**
- **Non-contrast CT**
- Hemorrhage(white)
- Ischemia (black)
- Carotid endarterectomy for symptomatic severe carotid stenosis >70 %

| Receptive(Wernicke) dysphasia | Expressive (Broca) dysphasia |
|---|---|
| - Temporal lobe (dominant side) <br> - Speak fluently but not meaningfully | - Frontal lobe (dominant side) <br> - Peak meaningfully but fluently |

### ❖ Horner syndrome:

- Idiopathic , Pancoast tumor , Internal carotid dissection , brainstem stroke/tumor
- Amyotrophic Lateral Sclerosis:(only motor system ,normal sensation)
- UMN+LMN palsy
- Normal sensation , bowel and bladder function
- Riluzole (treatment)

# Upper Limb Neurological Examination

❖ **Spinal cord lesions:**

| Anterior Cord Syndrome | Central Cord Syndrome | Posterior Cord Syndrome |
|---|---|---|
| • Corticospinal(UMN lesion signs) and spinothalamic tracts involved<br>• Bilateral loss of pain & temperature ,spastic muscle<br>• Dorsal column spared<br>• Anterior spinal infarction (AAA surgery) | • Syringomyelia | • Loss of proprioception and vibration (dorsal column)<br>• Due to : B12, tabless dorsalis ,Friedreich ataxia |

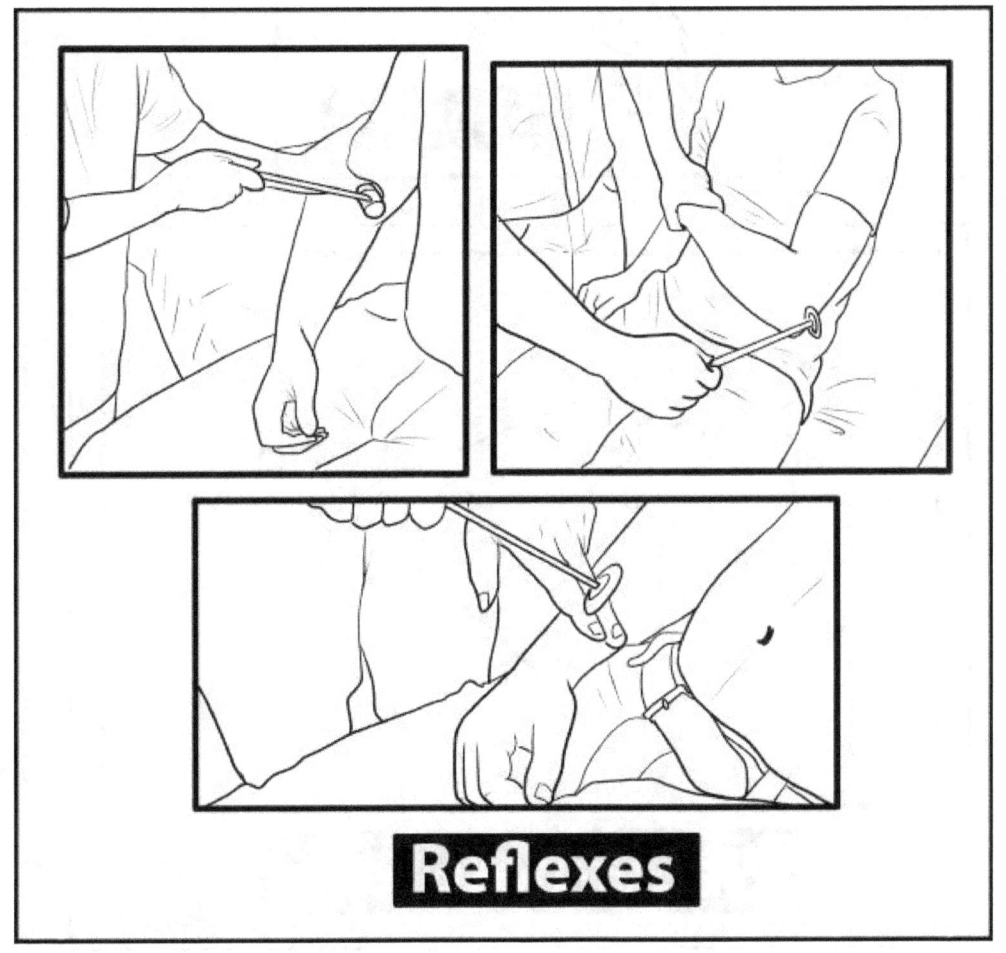

Reflexes

149

# Upper Limb Neurological Examination

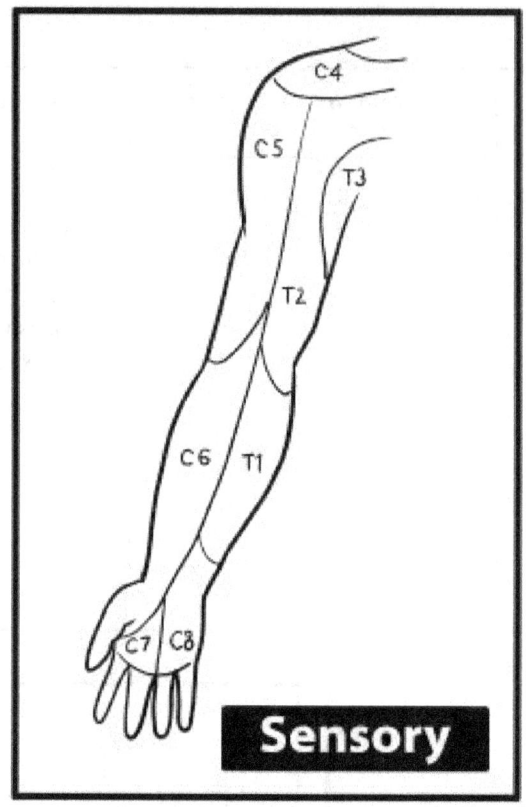

Sensory

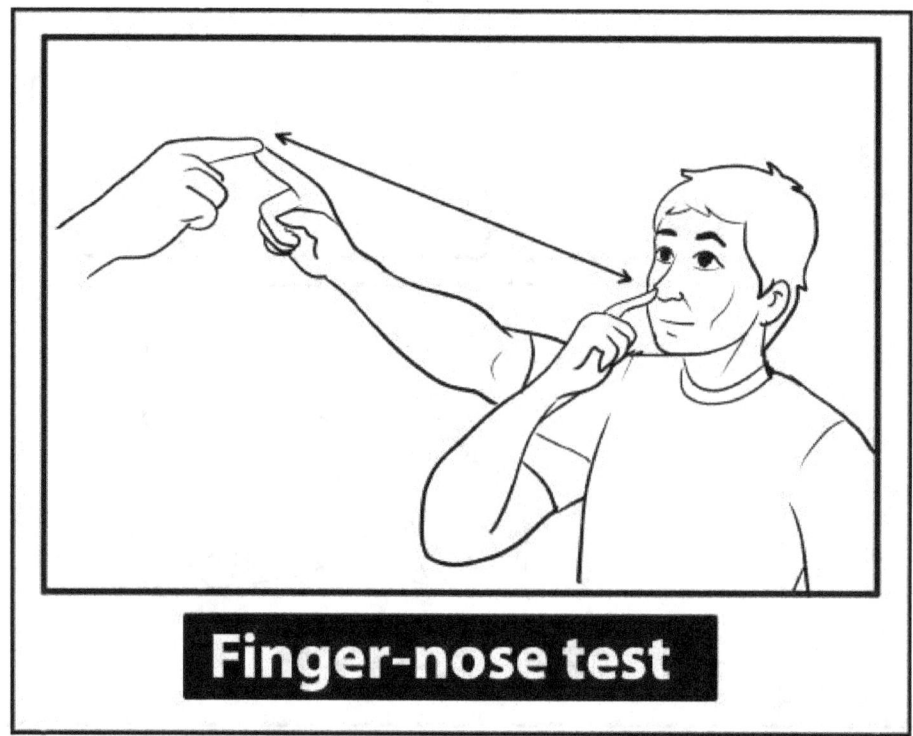

Finger-nose test

## Upper Limb Neurological Examination

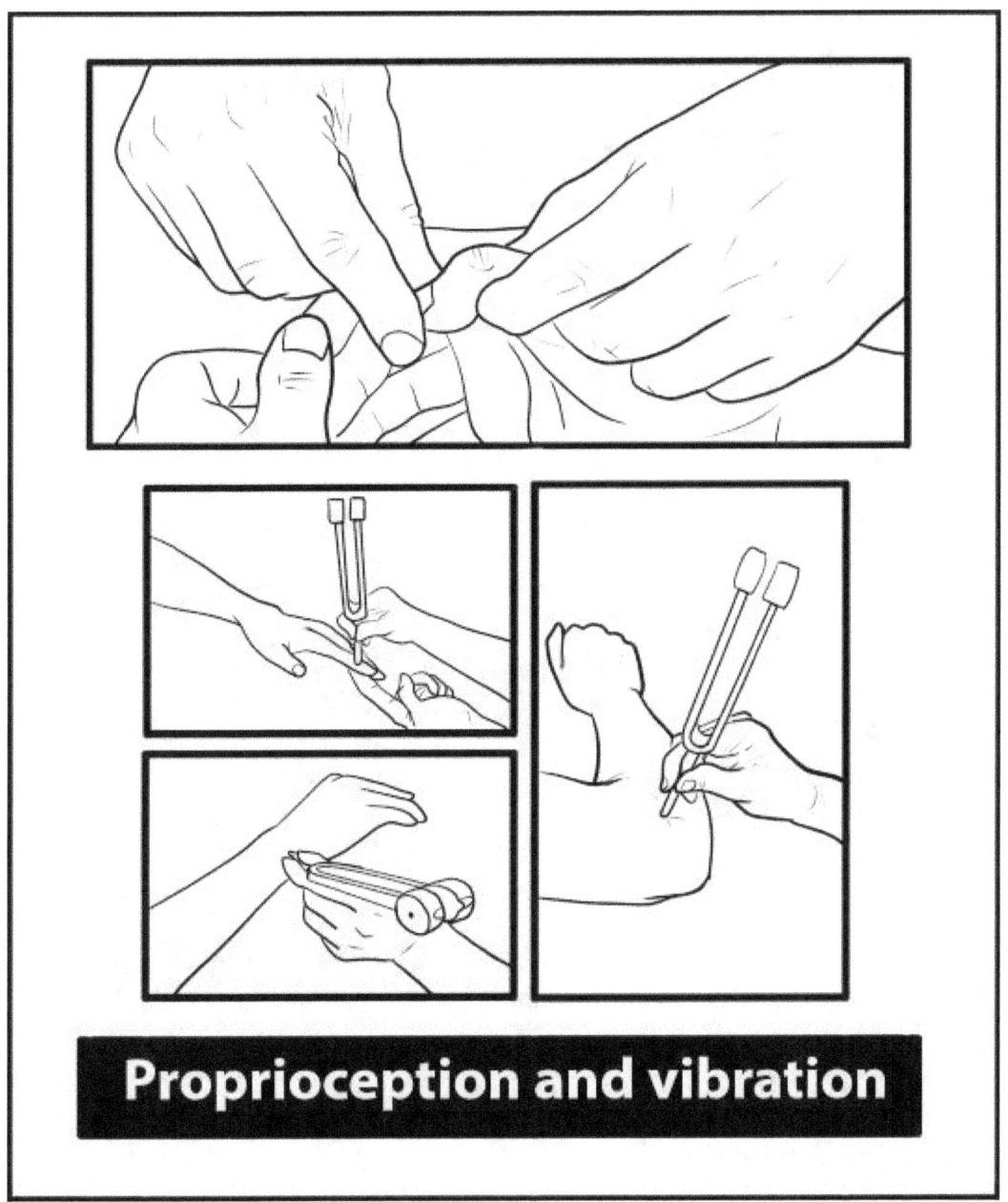

Proprioception and vibration

# Left cerebral lesion
## right sided findings

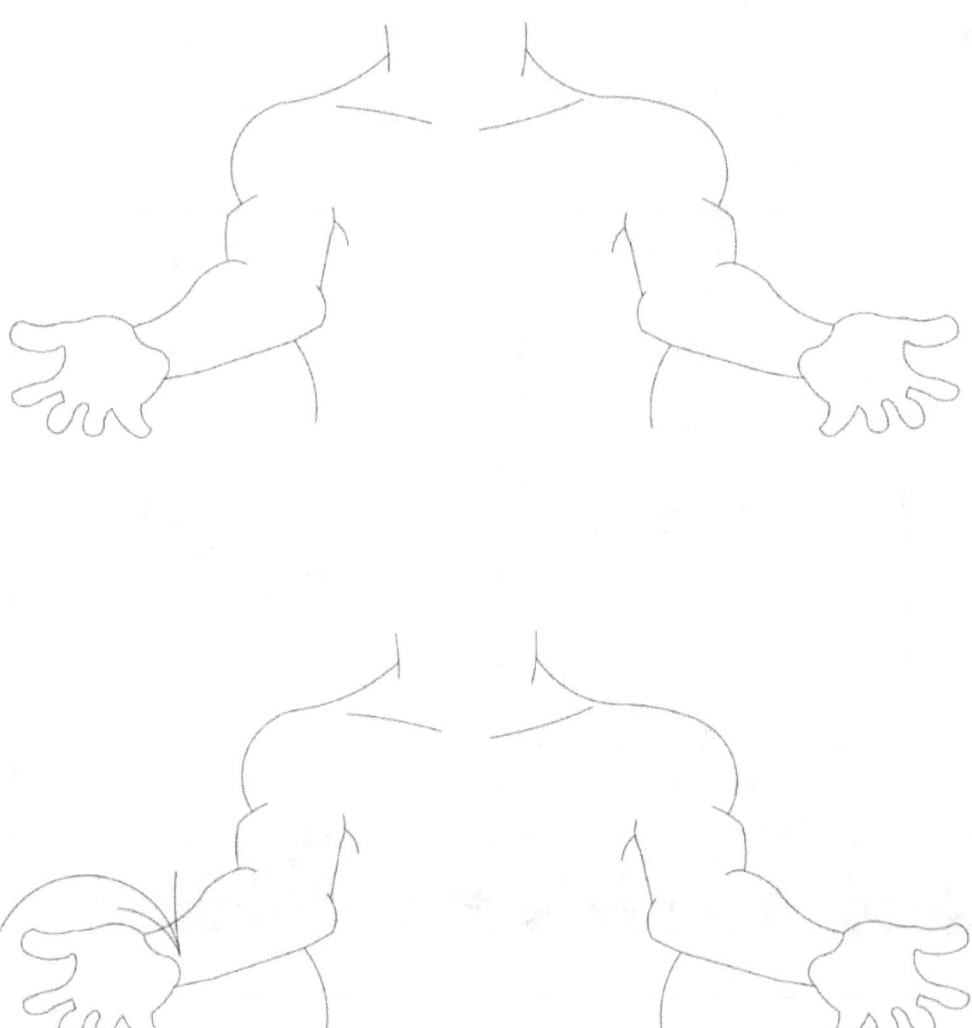

# Lower Limb Neurological Examination

| | |
|---|---|
| **General** | 1. Wash hands, introduce yourself, get name and age, explain your role out pain and gain permission<br>2. At 45 degrees, shorts only (legs exposed)<br>3. Always compare both legs<br>4. Around bed: drugs, Mobility Aids<br>5. Patient: posture, speech |
| **Inspection** | • Wasting, fasciculation,<br>• Asymmetry, deformity, scars<br>• Abnormal Position: hemiplegia (leg is extended and ankle, toes plantarflexed)<br>• Involuntary movements |
| **Tone** | • Floppy<br>• Hypertonia or hypotonia<br>• Rolling the thigh left and right repeatedly<br>• Sharply lift knee off the bed<br>* normally foot will not be lifted from bed, in hypertonia foot will be lifted<br>• Rule out ankle clonus (more than 3beats)<br>* UMNL |
| **Motor** | ▪ **Grade power in these movements with muscle isolation:**<br>• flexion, extension, abduction and adduction of hip<br>• flexion and extension of knee<br>• plantarflexion and dorsiflexion of ankle<br>• big toes extension |
| **Reflexes** | * **Maneuver to reinforce reflexes:** fingers looked and pulled apart<br>- Look at the muscle<br>• Knee reflex (L3, L4) (quadriceps)<br>• Ankle reflex (S1) (gastrocnemius muscle): both knee and ankle flexed at 90 degrees<br>• Babinski reflex or plantar response (L5, S1, S2)<br>* Positive UMNL =dorsiflexion of big toe |

## Lower Limb Neurological Examination

| | |
|---|---|
| **Co-ordination**<br>Cerebellar dysfunction | • Heel-shin test<br>• Foot tapping |
| **Standing** | • **Romberg's test (proprioception)**<br>• Be close in case patient falls<br>• Feet together and eye closed for 30 sec<br>• Positive =instability, loss of balance<br>• **Gait:**<br>• posture, balance, swinging of the arms, and movements of the legs<br>• broad-based gait (cerebellar ataxia)<br>• Shuffling gait (parkinson)<br>• Hemiplegic gait: circumduction<br>• high-stepping gait (foot drop)<br>To walk<br><br>- on heels (L4/L5)<br>- on tiptoes (S1/S2)<br>- heel-to-toe (cerebellar disease) |
| **The End** | • Anal reflex and saddle anaesthesia (cauda equina syndrome<br>• Straight-Leg raise test (L5, S1 disc herniation)<br>• Patient supine with extended leg<br>• Passively raise leg till 90 degrees no pain<br>• Positive = sciatica-like pain<br>• Cranial nerves and upper limb neurological examination |

## Lower Limb Neurological Examination

|  | Movement and muscle | Nerve |
|---|---|---|
| **Hip** | Flexion(Iliopsoas) | Iliofemoral nerve **(L1,2)** |
|  | Extension (Gluteus maximus) | Sciatic **(L5,S1)** |
| **Knee** | Flexion (Hamstrings) | Sciatic **(L5,S1)** |
|  | extension(Quadriceps) | Femoral **(L3,4)** |
| **Ankle** | Dorsiflexion (Tibialis anterior) | Deep peroneal **L4, L5** Foot drop |
|  | Plantar flexion(Gastrocnemius and soleus) | Tibial(S1/2) *Tarsal Tunnel Syndrome |
| **Great toe** | Dorsiflexion (Extensor hallucis longus) | Deep peroneal **(L5)** |

**_Diabetic foot_** :can present with **_neuropathic_** or **_ischemic_** features or **_both_**

-Clawing fingers

| Neuropathic | Ischemic |
|---|---|
| -Dry, warm pinky foot( normal pulses)  - Reduced sensation of pinprick, light touch and vibration sensation.  Absent of Achilles' reflex  -Ulcers is painless | - Shiny hairless cold foot(reduced pulses) - Ulcer is painful |

## Lower Limb Neurological Examination

|  | MS |
|---|---|
| **Clinical features** | - **Eye:**<br>  - INO (MLF syndrome)<br>  - Nystagmus<br>  - Diplopia<br>  - optic neuritis<br>- Scanning speech<br>- Uhthoff phenomenon<br>- Cerebellar dysfuction<br>- Autonomic dysfunction<br>- UMNL (mostly), LMNL, mixed<br>- Lhermitte sign<br>- Uhthoff's phenomenon (worsening of symptoms in hot climate or hot bath)<br>- Investigations:<br>  - CSF: immunoglobulin G, Oligoclonal bands<br>  - T2-weighted MRI |
| **Treatment** | - Methylprednisolone<br>- Beta-interferon<br>- Natalizumab<br>- Spasticity (baclofen)<br>- Tremor (buspirone)<br>- Cholinesterase inhibitor (urinary incontinence) |

❖ **Medical medullary syndrome**

### A. IPSILATERAL
1. XII[th] nerve palsy (tongue)

### B. CONTRALATERAL
1. Hemiplegia – sparing the face
2. Hemianesthesia sparing the face

# Lower Limb Neurological Examination

1. **Sciatica**:

    - Radicular shooting pain along the sciatic nerve distribution (buttock, thigh, leg, foot)
    - Worsened by coughing, sneezing
    - **LMNL:** lower limb weakness and flaccid paralysis
    - **Sensory:** numbness, paraesthesia
    - Reflexes losses

    - **Due:**
        - Compression
        - Disc herniation at L5, S1
        - Spinal stenosis, tumor, abscess, hematoma
        - lumbar spondylolisthesis
        - Pregnancy

    *straight leg raise test

2. **Cauda equina syndrome:**
    - Sciatica-like pain
    - Same clinical features of sciatica
    - Urinary, fecal retention and Incontinence
    - Impotence
    - Saddle anesthesia

    - **Due:**
    *lumbosacral nerves

    - Disc herniation
    - Spinal stenosis
    - Abscess, tumor, hematoma

3. **SCD (subacute combined degeneration):**
    - Due to b12 deficiency, pernicious anemia, terminal ileum disease(crohn)
    - bilateral loss of proprioception and vibration (dorsal column tract)
    - spastic muscle (corticospinal tract)
    - cerebellar sign

# Lower Limb Neurological Examination

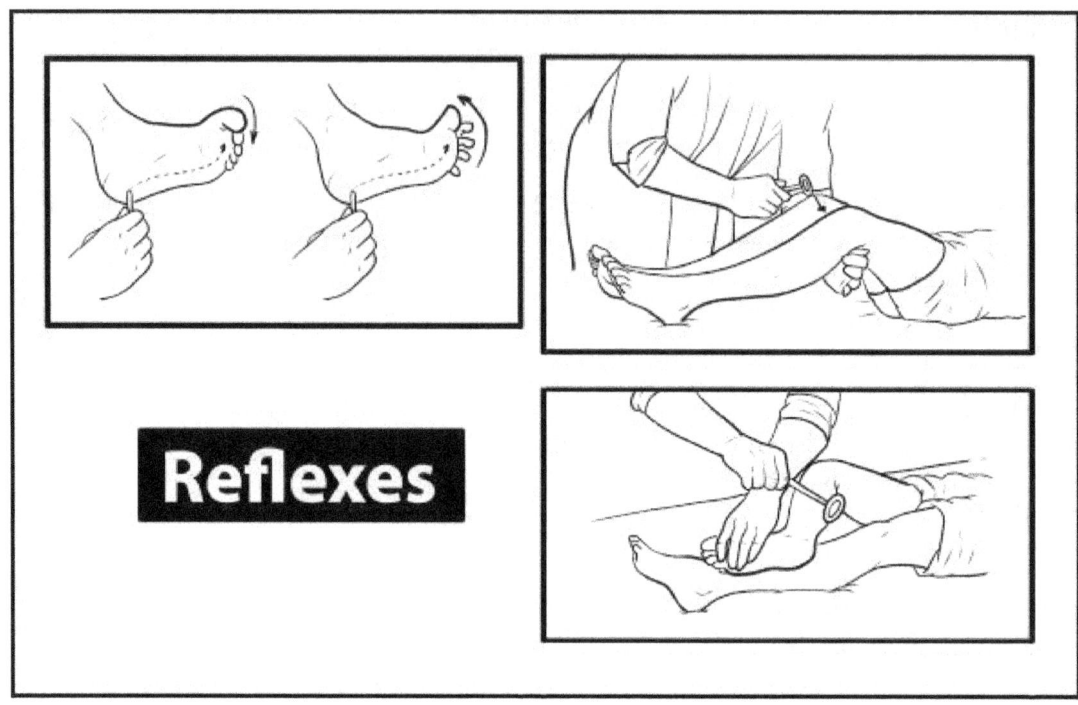

## Reflexes

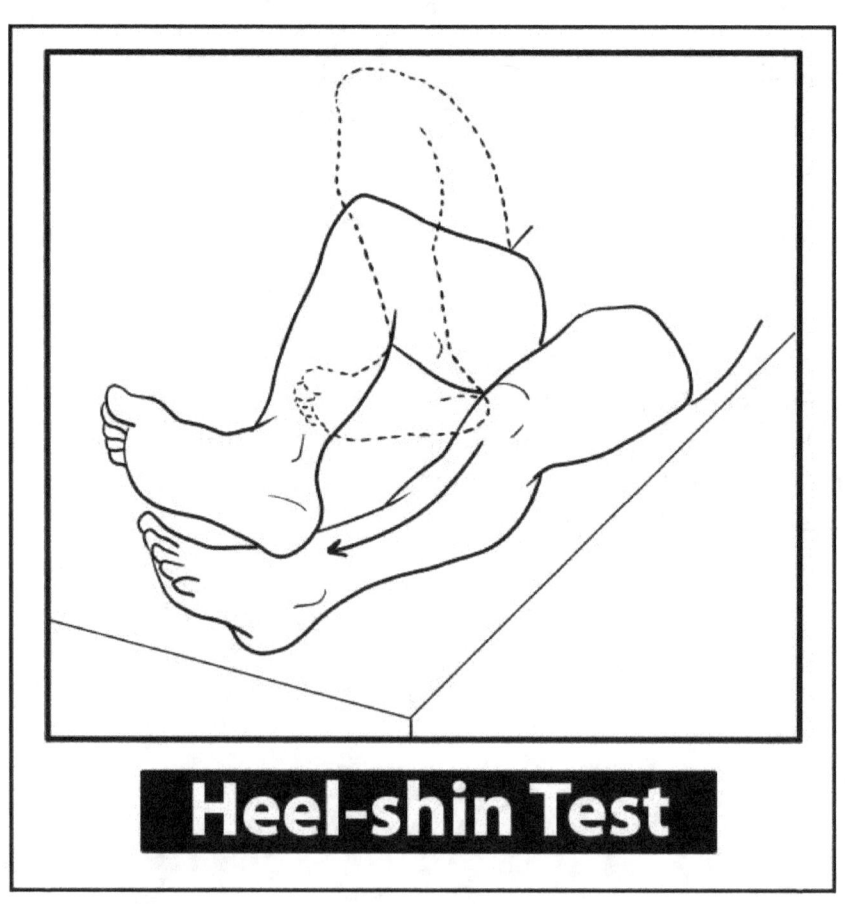

## Heel-shin Test

# Lower Limb Neurological Examination

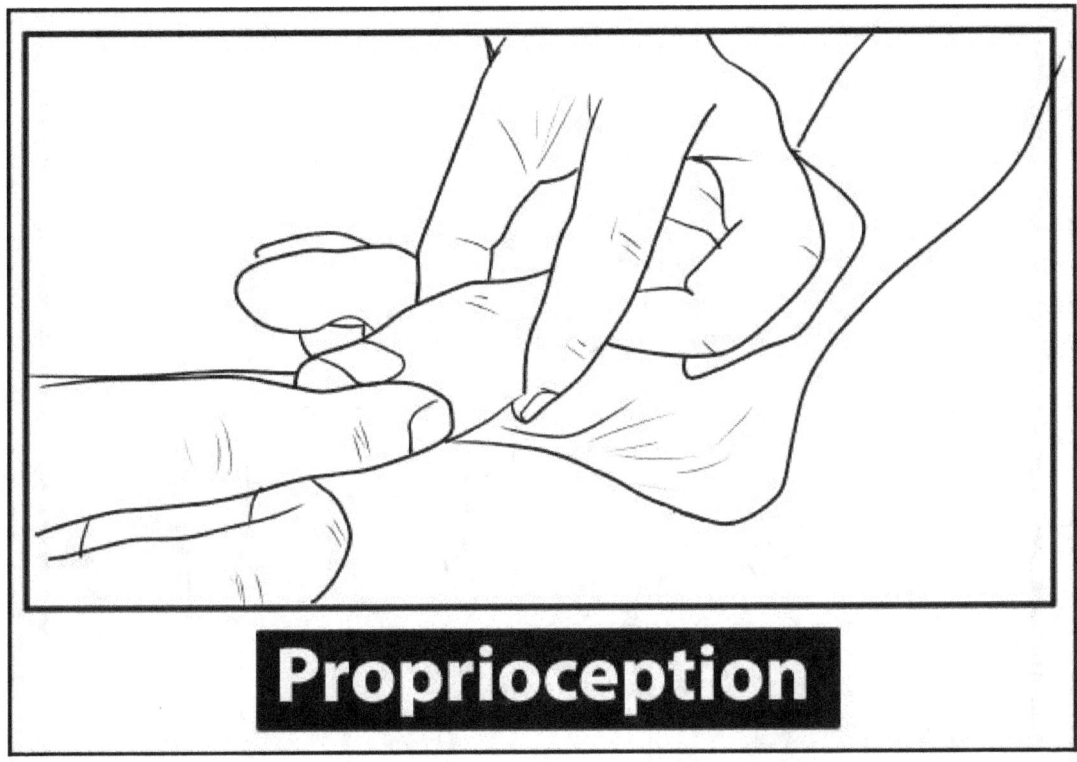

**Proprioception**

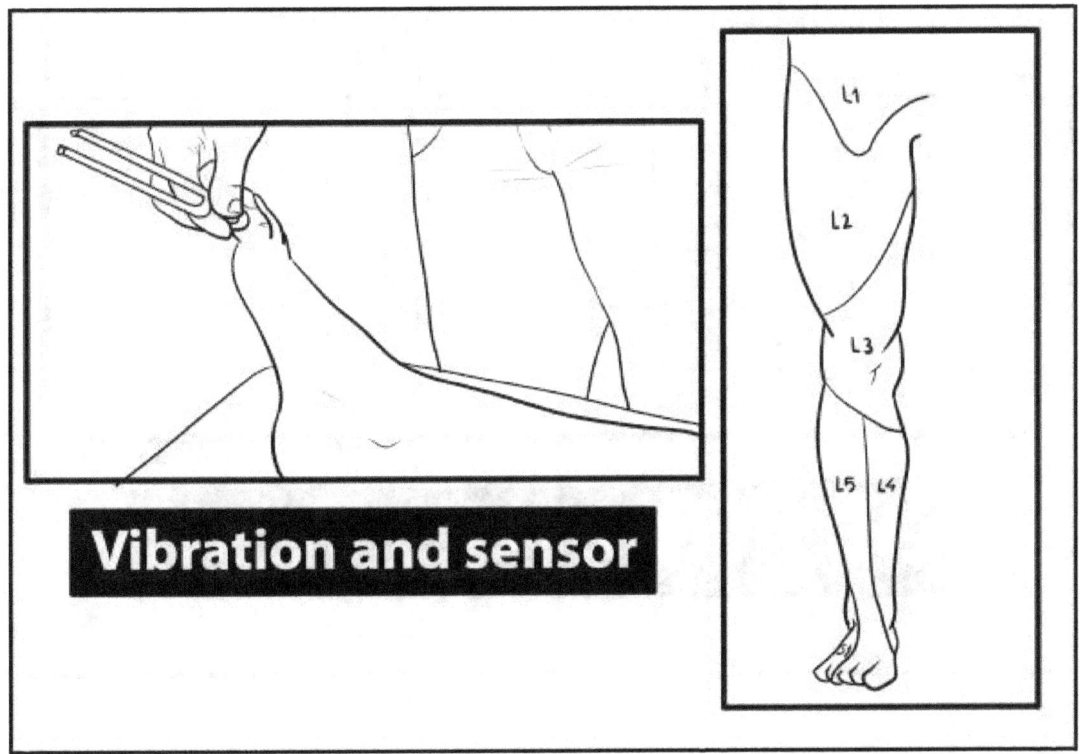

**Vibration and sensor**

# Lower Limb Neurological Examination

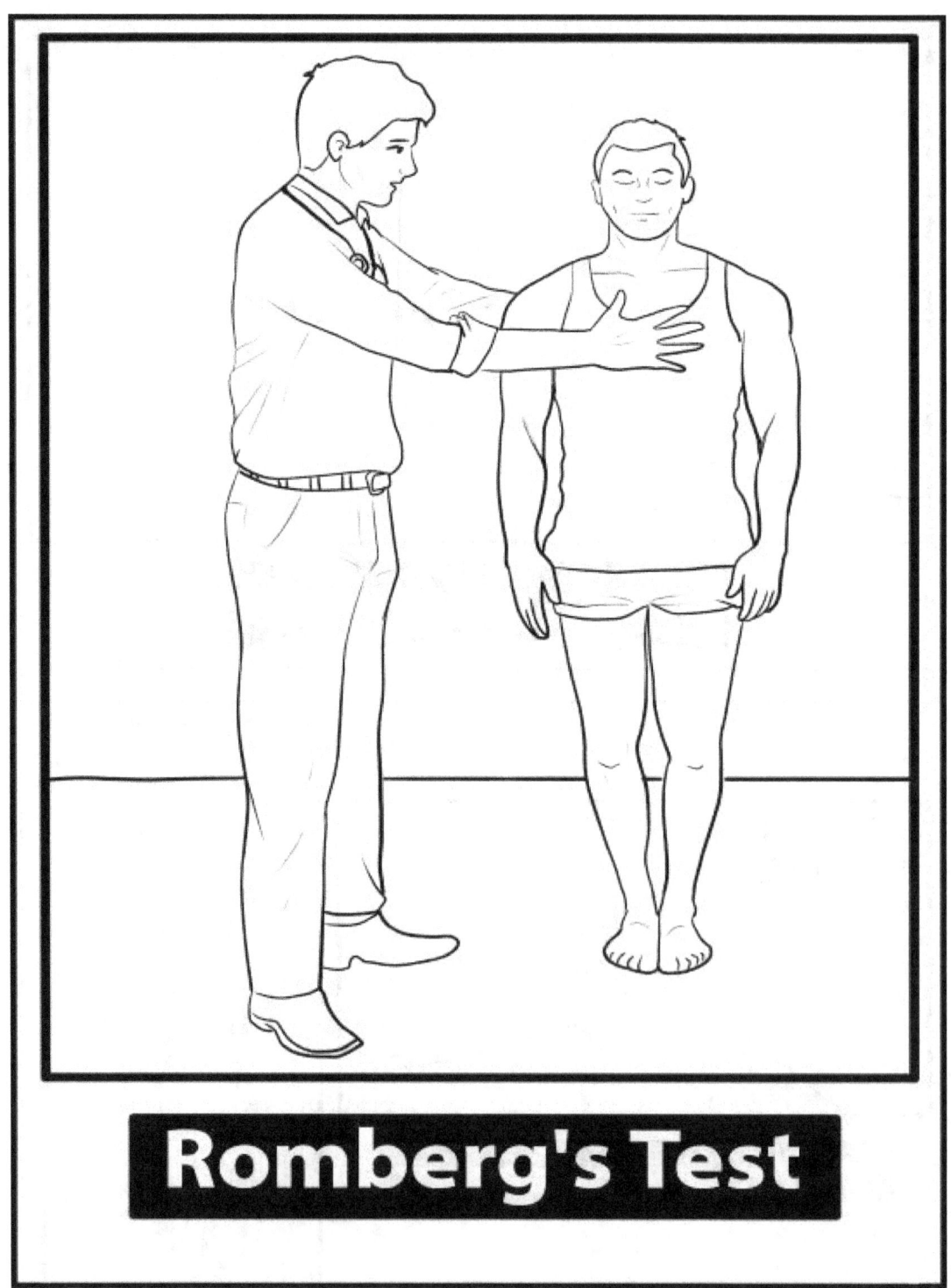

Romberg's Test

# Cranial Nerve Examination

| | |
|---|---|
| **General** | 1. Wash hands, introduce yourself, get name and age, explain your role out pain and gain permission<br>2. Sitting on a chair<br>3. Around bed (wheelchair, drugs)<br>4. Dominant hand |
| **CN1 Olfactory** | - Smell<br>- Anosmia due to skull tumors, fracture of cribriform plate of ethmoid |
| **CN2 Optic** | - **Visual acuity:** Snellen chart<br>- Examine both eyes (lenses, eyeglasses must be worn)<br>- One eye covered<br>- Read letters from top to below 6m away<br>**\*if unable to read any of letters move 3 meters and do it again, move 1 meter, if he can count fingers on your hand, move your hand and ask if he can see it, any light from the room**<br><br>- **Visual Field:** Without wearing glasses<br>- Sit directly facing the patient, knees opposite to Pt knees, your chest is about 1 meter away from his chest.<br>- Ask the patient to keep looking at your nose<br>- Patient covers one eye (examiner cover the same side eye), the examined eye focus in your nose<br>- Hold your hand halfway between you and the Pt<br>- Move your fingers in from peripheries to center (2,4,8,10 o'clock) X shape<br>- Pathway (retina -optic n-optic chiasm-optic tract-LGN-two pathways Meyer loop and dorsal optic radiation-Calcarine fissure<br>- **Lesions:**<br>a. **Scotoma:** (macular degeneration) central vision loss (peripheral fine)<br>b. **Right or left anopia** (optic nerve disorder (neuritis)<br>c. **Optic chiasm:** bitemporal hemianopia (pituitary tumor)<br>d. **Optic tract:** homonymous hemianopia<br>\* Lesion on contralateral side of brain<br>e. **Meyer loop:** upper quadrantanopia (contralateral temporal tumor, MCA infarction)<br>f. **Dorsal optic radiation:** lower quadrantanopia (parietal tumor, MCA infarction<br>g. **Calcarine fissure:** hemianopia with macular sparing (PCA infarction) |

# Cranial Nerve Examination

- **Pupillary light reaction(CN2,3):** PERRLA (pupils equal, round, and reactive to light and accommodation
- **Pathway:** retina-optic nerve-pretectal nuclei activate both Edinger Westphal
  - Nuclei activate both CN3 to constrict both pupils
- The pupillary light reaction
  - **Afferent:** optic nerve.
  - **Efferent:** parasympathetic component of the third nerve on both sides.
  a. Direct reflex (shine light onto the affected while looked at the wall).
  b. Consensual reflex: (look at the contralateral pupil should constrict).
  - If dilated pupil react to light and accommodate t (normal).
  - Dilated pupil does not react to light + but accommodate (afferent pupillary defect)
  - Dilated pupil that neither react nor accommodate (CN3 palsy)
  - Small pupil that react to the light and accommodate (horner syndrome)
  - Bilateral Small pupils that does not react to light but accommodate (Argyll Robertson pupil)
- **Light swinging test:** shine light for 1 sec between two eyes RAPD (marcus gunn pupil)
  1. when light is shined into diseased eye it remains dilated and the healthy eye is dilated
  2. Now shine the light onto the healthy eye, both the healthy and diseased eyes are constricted
  - accommodation response (constriction, convergence)
  - While patient looked at wall, then ask patient to focus on your finger
- **Accommodation reaction**
  - **Afferent:** frontal lobes.
  - **Efferent:** CN 3

- Amsler grid(scotoma)
- Visual inattention (Hemispatial neglect)
- Colour vision
- Blind spot (central scotoma)

- **Fundoscopy:**
  - Papilledema (swollen optic disc)

- **Pathology:**

# Cranial Nerve Examination

| | |
|---|---|
| | 1. Afferent pupillary defect: anterior to optic chiasm Like retinal diseases, optic nerve compression by tumor, aneurysm, optic neuritis.<br>2. Relative afferent pupillary defect(RAPD) same as above<br>3. Argyll–Robertson pupil: DM, syphilis, midbrain lesion |
| **CN 3,4,5**<br><br>**Oculomotor, Trochlear, and Abducens** | - Sitting in chairs in front of each other:<br>- Inspect ptosis, squint<br>- Comment on head position: head is tilted away from the side of lesion (CN4 palsy)<br>- **Eye movement:** H pattern<br>- Look nystagmus, conjugate movements<br>- Ask for pain, diplopia<br>- head still<br>- Just eyes are moving<br>- If Pt has double vision: You have to know the CN/muscle and the eye affected<br>- Ask which direction its maximum widest apart (this tells you the CN/muscle)<br>- Ask the Pt to cover the one eye<br>- If the outer image disappears<br>- Then this is the affected eye and the closed eye is the false<br>\* Diplopia at lateral direction (CN6 palsy),<br>\* Downward and medially to nose (CN4 palsy)<br>\* Other directions can be caused by:<br>a. Thyroid grave diseases<br>b. Variable ptosis (worsen by end of day, improve by applying ice cube on it):MG<br>c. Eye down and out +/-constant ptosis CN3 palsy<br>1. dilated pupil =Posterior communicating aneurysm<br>2. Normal pupil =DM<br><br>▪ **DD of diplopia:**<br>- CN palsy<br>- NMJ (myasthenia gravis)<br>- Muscle disease<br><br>● **Damaged:**<br>- CN3(MR+SR+IR+IO) and upper eyelid<br>  Eye down and out, unresponsive to light +ptosis Due to PCA, DM<br><br>- CN4(SO)<br>  Eye is upward, head tilted away from lesion side head trauma<br>- CN6(LR) |

# Cranial Nerve Examination

| | |
|---|---|
| | Eye is inward(abducted)<br><br>• **MR** (medially)<br>• **LR**(laterally)<br>• **SO** (inferomedially)<br>• **IO**(superomedially)<br>• **SR**(superolaterally)<br>• **IR**(inferolaterally)<br><br>• **Internuclear ophthalmoplegia(INO):**<br>- MLF lesions due (MS, pons infarction)<br>- MLF connects CN6 nucleus on one side with the CN3 nucleus on the opposite side of the brainstem<br>• **Lesion:** ipsilateral paralysis of adduction and the contralateral nystagmus<br>* **Ptosis (Horner's syndrome, CN3 palsy, MG, injury)** |
| **CN5**<br><br>**Trigeminal** | • **Sensory:**<br>• with neurotip & cotton<br>• Eyes closed (test on sternum)<br>• On each sides:<br>a. forehead (ophthalmic N V1)<br>b. cheeks (maxillary N V2)<br>c. Jaw (mandibular N V3)<br>• **Motor:**<br>• palpating the temporal and masseter muscles while patient clenching teeth (atrophy)<br>• resist Jew opening (pterygoid muscle)<br>* **jaw will deviate to side of lesion**<br>• **Offer to do**<br>• Jaw jerk: brisk occurs in UMN<br>• Corneal Reflex. Blinking CN5 specifically V1 (afferent) to CN7(efferent) |
| **CN 7 Facial** | • **Inspection:**<br>- **External auditory meatus**: Herpes zoster oticus (Ramsay Hunt syndrome)<br>- **Hyperacusis:** stapedius muscle paralysis (hearing loud noises)<br>- Asymmetry<br><br><br>- Loss of Forehead wrinkles, flattening of the nasolabial fold, drooping of the corner mouth |

# Cranial Nerve Examination

|  |  |
|---|---|
|  | - **Bell's phenomenon:** upward movement of eye on attempt to close it<br><br>- **Movements:**(asymmetry)<br>- Raise both eyebrows(Frontalis)<br>- Close both eyes tightly (try to open it=strength) Orbicularis oculi<br>- Show both upper and lower teeth (smile) (Buccinators)<br>- Puff out both cheeks (place your fingers =strength) (Orbicularis oris)<br>a. **UMNL:**<br>- contralateral facial paralysis (forehead preserved)<br>  Stroke, MS, tumor<br><br>b. **LMN:**<br>- Ipsilateral facial paralysis (forehead affected)<br>Cannot raise forehead and close eye<br><br>- Hyperacusis<br>- Loss of taste ⅔ anterior tongue<br>**Due:** HIV, sarcoidosis & GBS (bilateral CN 7 palsy), Lyme, lesions at the cerebellopontine angle, parotid (tumor, surgery), bell's palsy*<br><br>* **Bell's palsy (LMN lesion)**<br>- **Risk Factors:** pregnant, DM, herpes simplex, herpes zoster (ramsay-hunt syndrome)<br>- **Cavernous sinus thrombosis:**<br>  (associated, III, IV, V1, VI) |
| **CN 8 Acoustic** | - Cover one ear and rub your fingers on the other ear (if its reduced do weber and rinne)<br>- **Or** whisper a number then ask patient to repeat it<br>- Air and bone conduction **(512Hz fork)**<br><br>- **Rinne Test:**<br>- Start in bone conduction **(mastoid)** then on beside ear **(air conduction)**<br><br>- Ask which one is louder?<br>* **Normal or Neural deafness:** air conduction > bone conduction<br>* **Conductive Deafness:** bone conduction > air conduction |

# Cranial Nerve Examination

|  |  |
|---|---|
|  | ▪ Weber Test<br>● Place on midline of forehead<br>● Ask if it is louder on the middle or more on one ear?<br>∗ **Neural Deafness:** lateralization away from affected ear<br>▪ **Conduction**<br>∗ **Normal:** on middle<br>∗ **Conductive:** more to the affected ear<br><br>▪ **Causes of Conductive Deafness:**<br>a. External ear pathology: foreign body, wax, tympanic membrane rupture<br>b. middle ear pathology: Osteoclerosis<br>  Otitis media<br>▪ **Sensorineural Deafness:**<br>● Age<br>- cochlea pathology: Ménière's disease, gentamicin, furosemide, noise<br>- CN8 palsy : meningitis, CPA tumours, MS.<br>- Pons pathology : vascular ,tumor |
| **CN 9-10 Glossopharyngeal and Vagus** | ▪ **Inspection:**<br>● Hoarseness (unilateral RLN) + nasal voice + strider (bilateral RLN)<br>● Open mouth notice uvula<br>∗ **Normally midline not deviated**<br>● Then ask to say ahh<br>∗ **Normally uvula will raise centrally upward and soft palate raise symmetrical**<br><br>▪ **Offer to do**<br>● **Water test:** drink water: choking, regurgitation through nose are indicative for CN 9& 10 palsy<br>● **Gag reflex** (both afferent CN9, efferent CN10)<br>∗ **Bilateral lesion CN 10 palate fails to raise**<br>∗ **Unilateral CN 10 lesions:** asymmetry palatal arch, uvula pulled toward the normal side (away from lesion) |
|  | - Shirt off<br>▪ **inspection**:<br>● trapezius and SCM for atrophy, fasciculation<br>▪ **Movements**:<br>- First without resistant then with resistance |

## Cranial Nerve Examination

| CN11<br>Spinal accessory<br>(Cervical nerves 1–5) | • shrug shoulders<br>• SCM: turn your head to left against resistant while your other hand feeling the right SCM<br>* **Left SCM will turn the head to the right**<br>* SCM: tilt the head to ipsilateral side, and rotate the head to contralateral side |
|---|---|
| CN 12<br>Hypoglossal N | ▪ **Comment on:**<br>• Speech, ask about any difficulties with swallowing<br>• Tongue:<br>a. **Opened mouth (inside mouth):** atrophy, fasciculation<br>b. **On protrusion:** deviation<br>- Lick it from side to side<br>- Push from inside of cheek while your fingers on Patient<br>- cheeks: weakness 9<br>* **LMN lesion:** ipsilateral weakness, atrophy, fasciculation, deviation toward to side of lesion<br>* **UMN lesions (usually bilateral):** bilateral weakness, spastic paralysis (cannot protrude it) |

1. **Bulbar palsy:** LMN palsy of cranial nerves 9,10,11,12 due ALS, MS, brainstem tumor/stroke, MG, GBS, MND
- Normal facial expression and jaw reflex
- Loss of gag reflex
- Tongue (wasting, fasciculation)


2. **Pseudobulbar palsy:** UMN palsy of CN 9,10,11,12 +5,7 due to Stroke, ALS, MS
- Loss Facial expression (CN7)
- Jaw reflex(brisk)
- Spastic tongue (difficulty to protrusion)
- Gag reflex (high, exaggerated)
- Emotional lability
* Both bulbar and pseudobulbar causes regurgitation, dysphagia (CN 10)


▪ **Causes of pupil dilation:**
a. CN3 palsy
- compression by PCA aneurysm (causing down and out eye + fixed and dilated pupil)
- Antimuscarinic eye drops
- Holmes Adie pupil: associated Hyporeflexia (Achilles tendon)

# Cranial Nerve Examination

- **Causes of pinpoint pupil:**
  - Opioid
  - Horner syndrome (ptosis, anhidrosis, miosis)

- **Causes of ptosis:**
1. **Unilateral:**
   - CN3 palsy, Horner's syndrome, MG

2. **Bilateral:**
   - MG, Myotonic dystrophy

- **Causes of Sensory Neuropathy:**
  - DM
  - Alcoholism
  - B12 deficiency
  - Chronic renal failure

- **Motor Neuropathy:**
  - GBS
  - Lead toxicity
  - Mononeuritis multiplex is a painful, asymmetrical, asynchronous sensory and motor peripheral neuropathy involving isolated damage to at least 2 separate nerve areas:
    - DM
    - Vasculitis/Wegener's granulomatosis /PAN
    - Amyloidosis

- **Alcohol CNS Complication:**
  - Sensory neuropathy
  - Wernicke-korsakoff syndrome:
  a. **Wernicke**(acute)
  - Ophthalmoplegia, nystagmus, confusion, ataxia
  b. **korsakoff**(chronic)
  - Confabulation (answers are not related to the question), amnesia
  - Cerbellar degeneration

- **Wallenberg Syndrome (lateral medullary syndrome):**
  - Posterior inferior cerebellar artery (PICA) infarction
  - Ipsilateral Horner's syndrome
  - Ipsilateral Cerebellar signs
  - Ipsilateral V (ipsilateral loss of pain and temperature over face)
  - IX (loss of gag reflex)
  - X (palatal paralysis, dysphagia)
  - XI (weak SCM)
  - Contralateral
  - Contralateral spinothalamic signs (loss of pain & temperature over body)

# Cranial Nerve Examination

- **Cerebellopontine Angle:**
- Benign schwannoma (unilateral)
- Neurofibromatosis type II(bilateral)
- **Nerves Involved:**
a. CN VIII (SNHL, Tinnitus)
b. CN V (ipsilateral facial numbness)

- **Myasthenia Gravis:**
- NMJ disease
- Autoantibodies to AChR
- Symptoms are improved by rest and worsen with the use of muscle (fatigue)
- Mostly involve:
- facial muscle (ptosis, dysphagia, dysarthria, diplopia)
- **Respiratory failure if diaphragm is involved**
- Ask Pt to count from 1 to 30
- There will be decrease of phonation as Pt reach 30
- Check Pt shoulder abduction power
- Then ask Pt move his arm up and down 20 times
- Then recheck the power again if its decreased then (positive)

- **Investigation**
- Acetylcholine receptor antibody test, CT (thymoma), Edrophonium test (Symptoms improvement)
- Treated by
- Pyridostigmine,
- Thymectomy
- Corticosteroids

# Cranial Nerve Examination

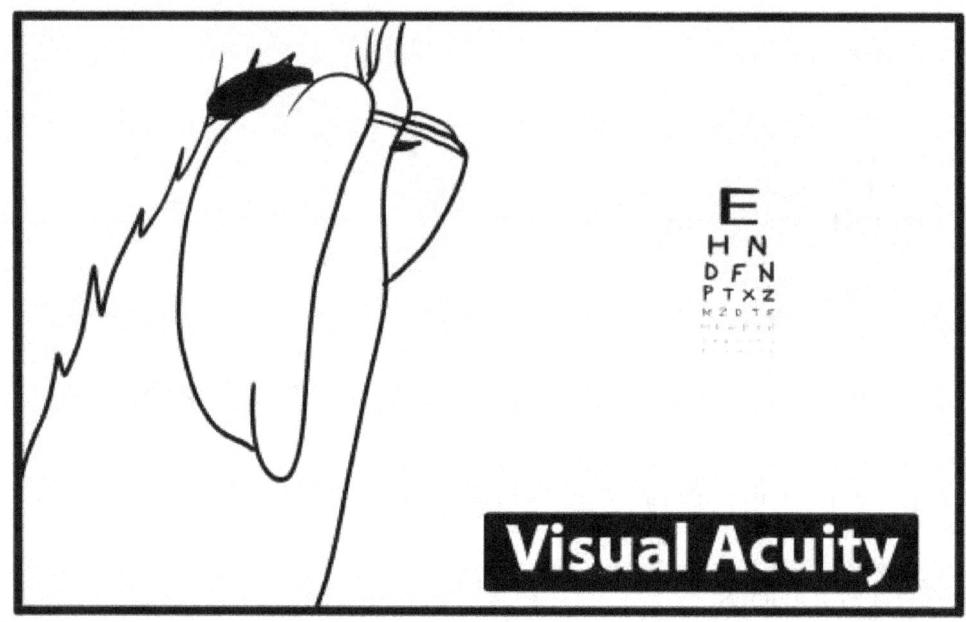

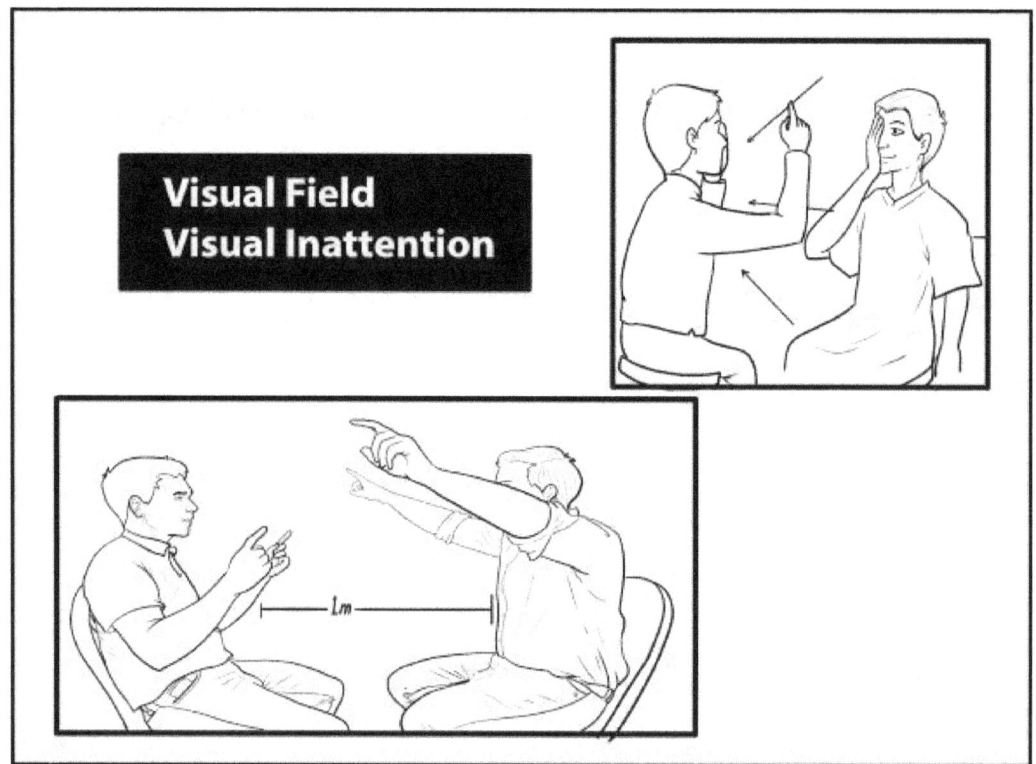

# Cranial Nerve Examination

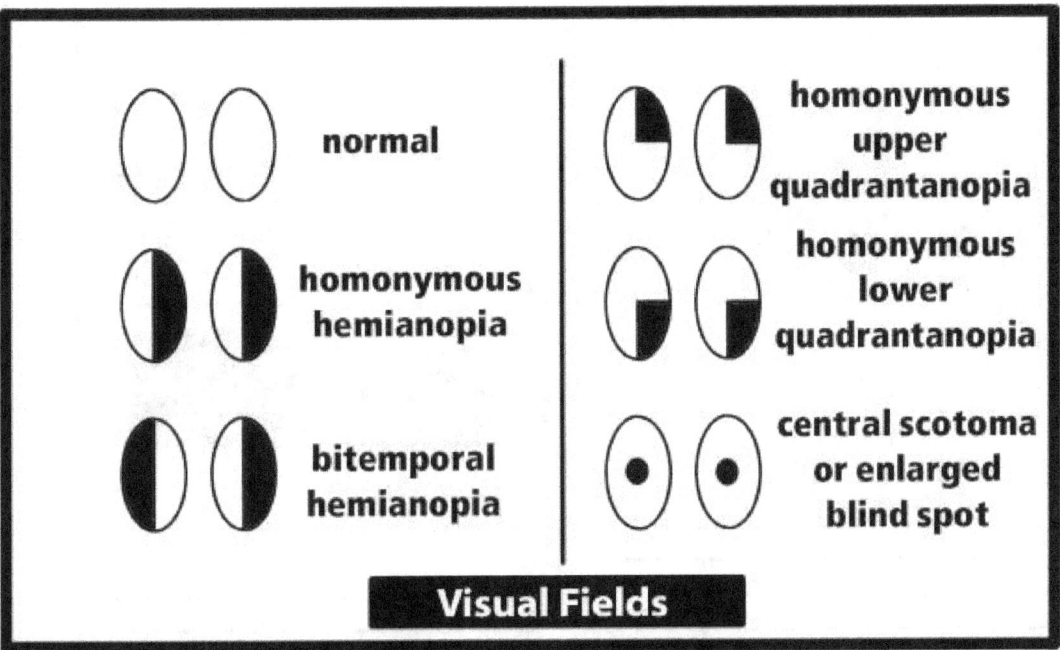

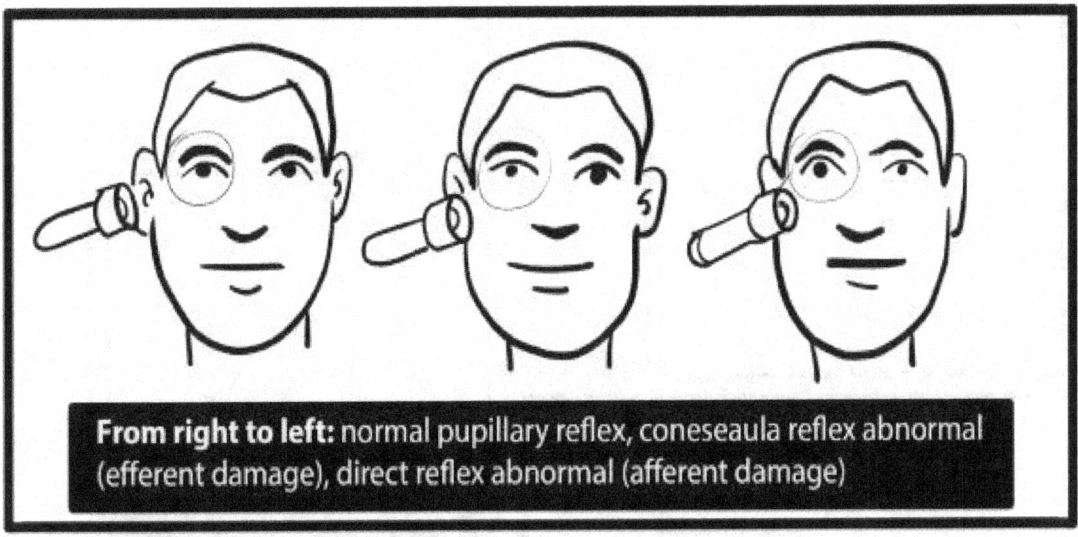

**From right to left:** normal pupillary reflex, coneseaula reflex abnormal (efferent damage), direct reflex abnormal (afferent damage)

# Cranial Nerve Examination

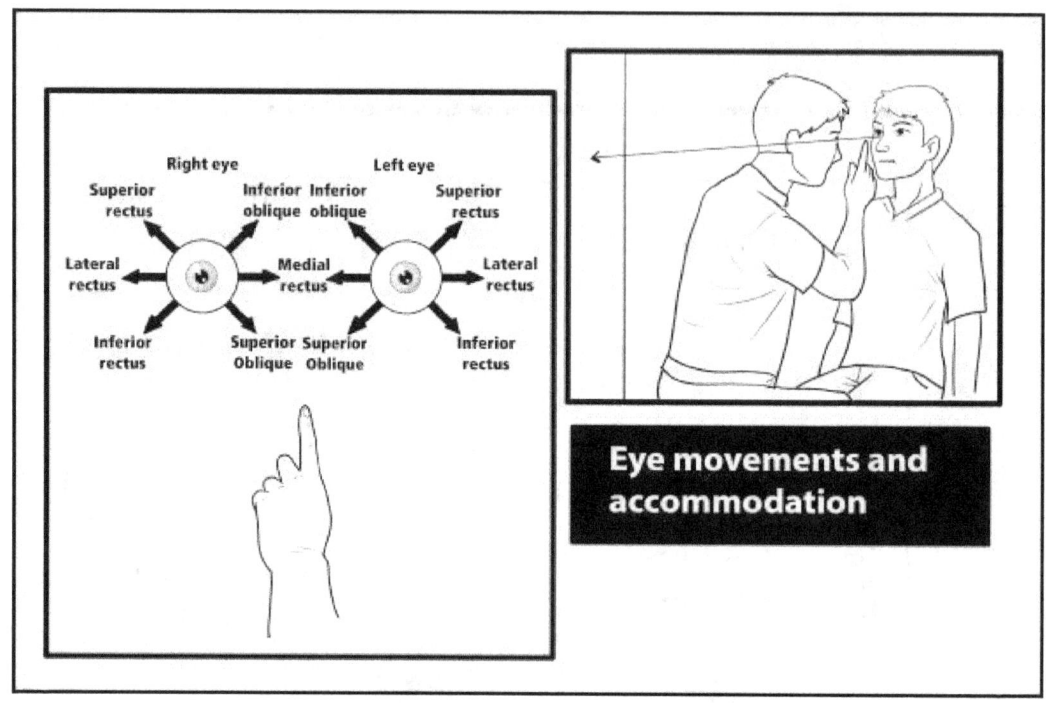

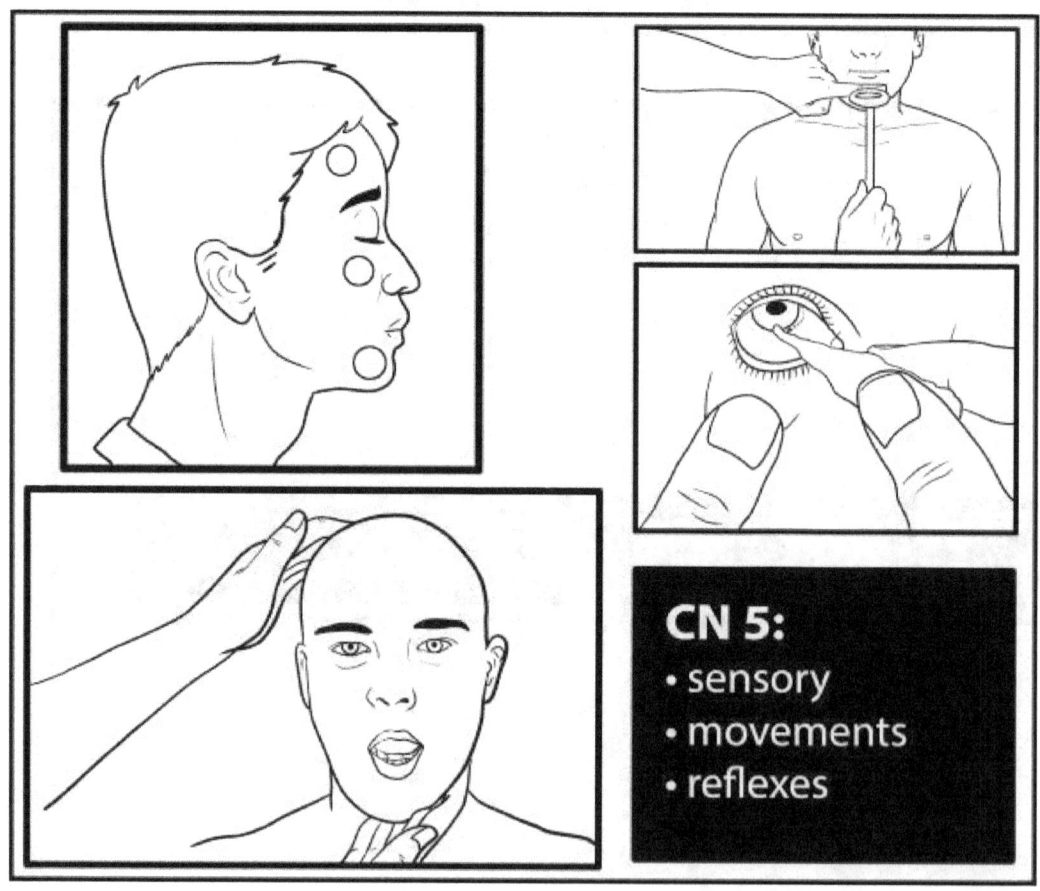

# Cranial Nerve Examination

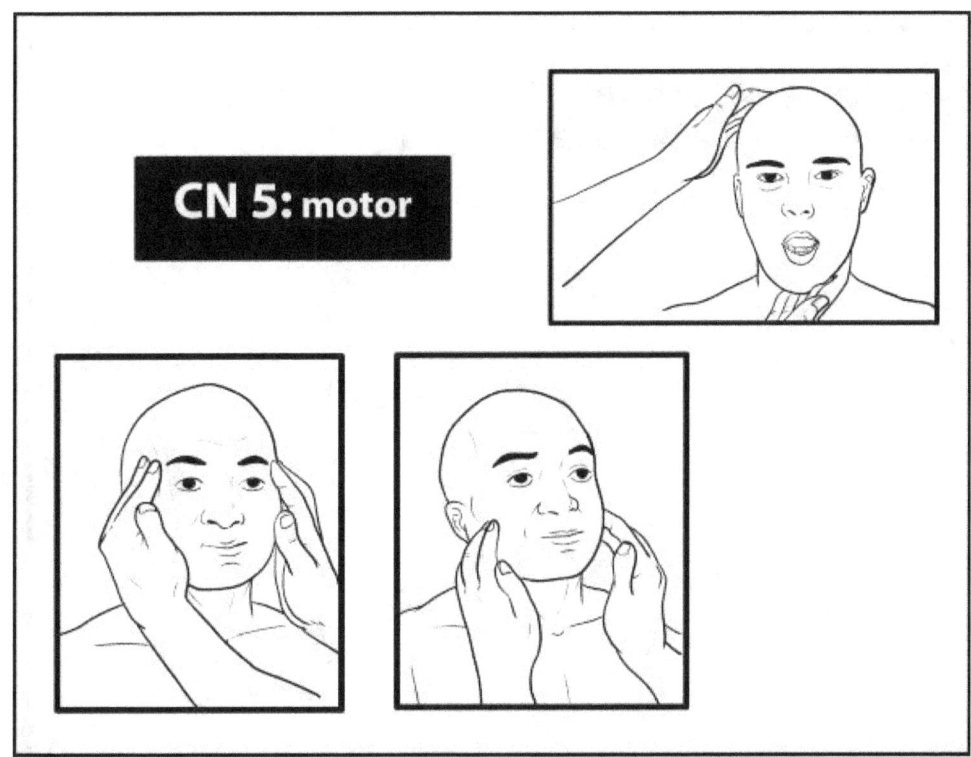

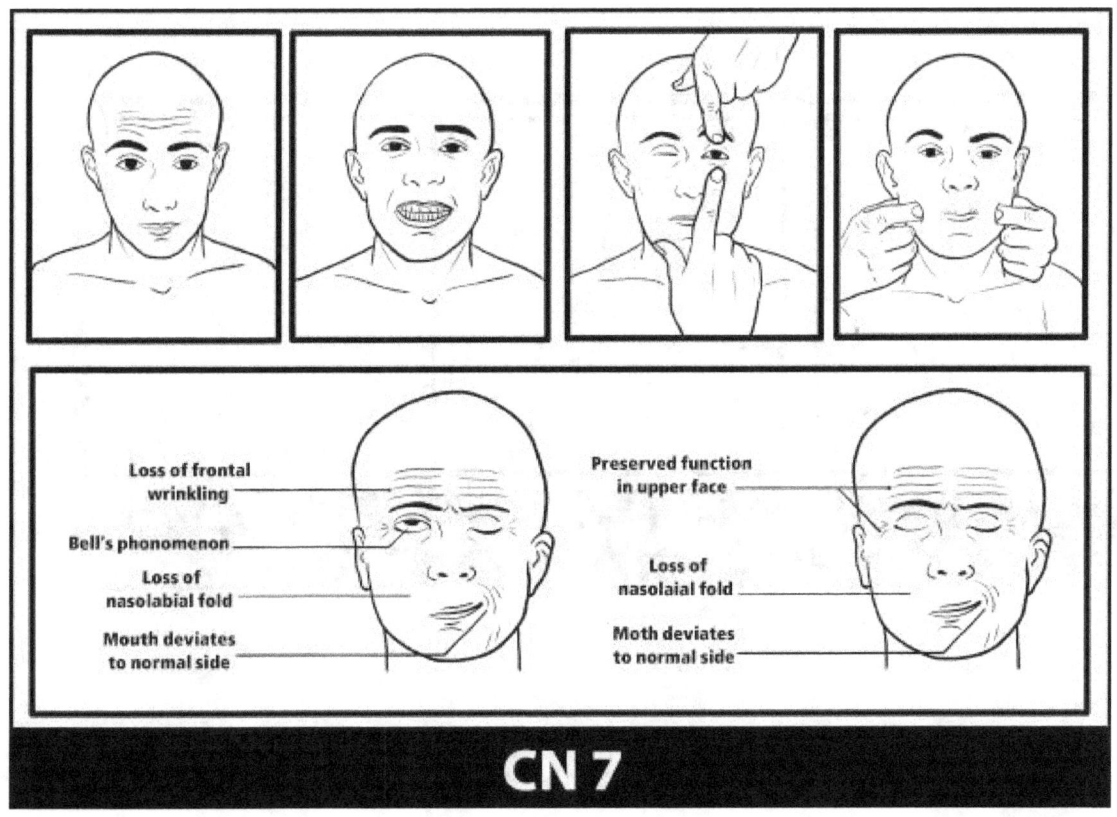

# Cranial Nerve Examination

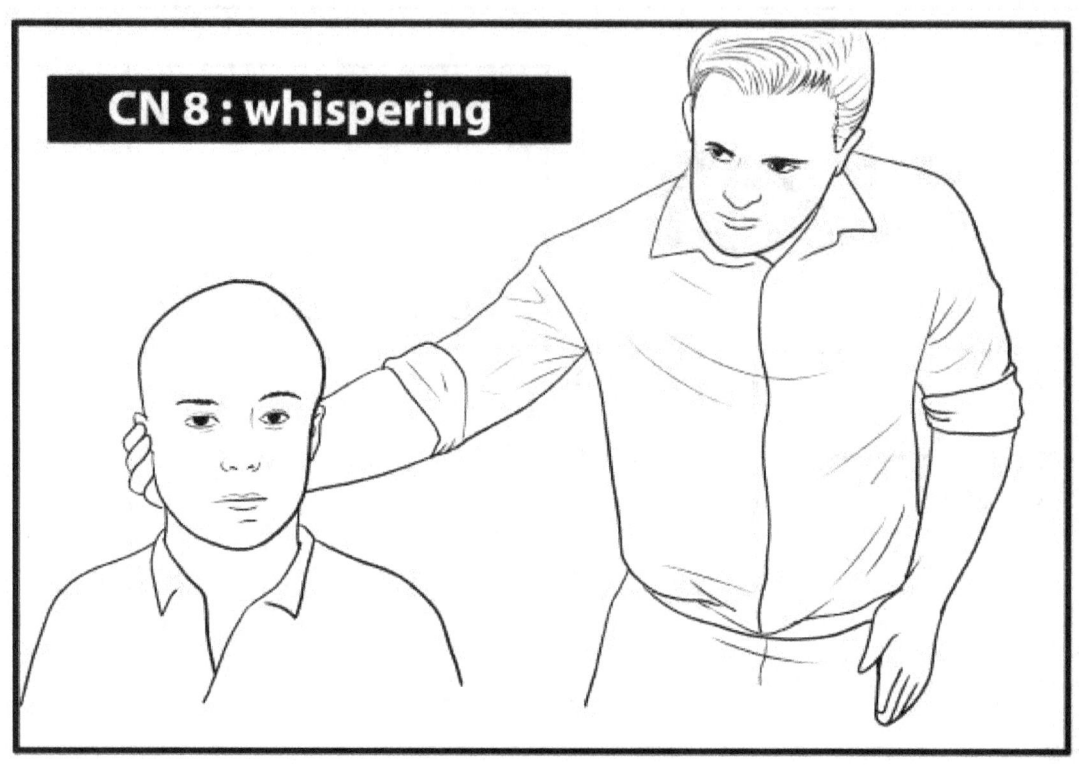

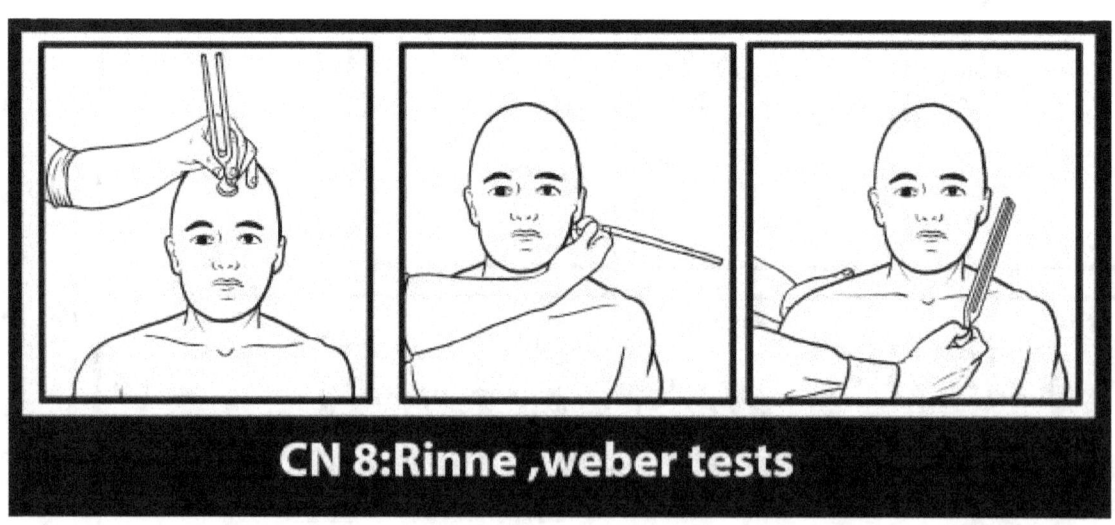

# Cranial Nerve Examination

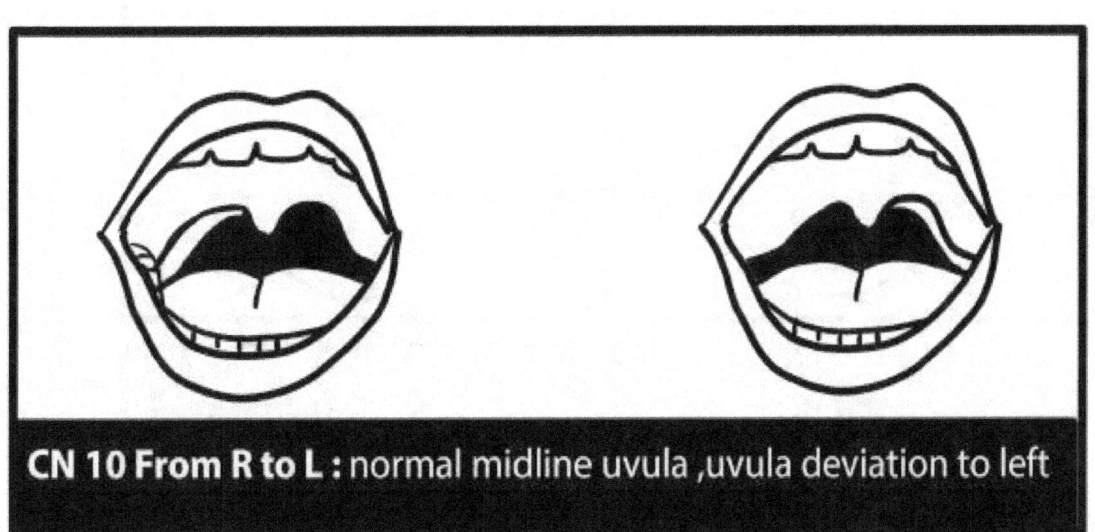

CN 10 From R to L : normal midline uvula, uvula deviation to left

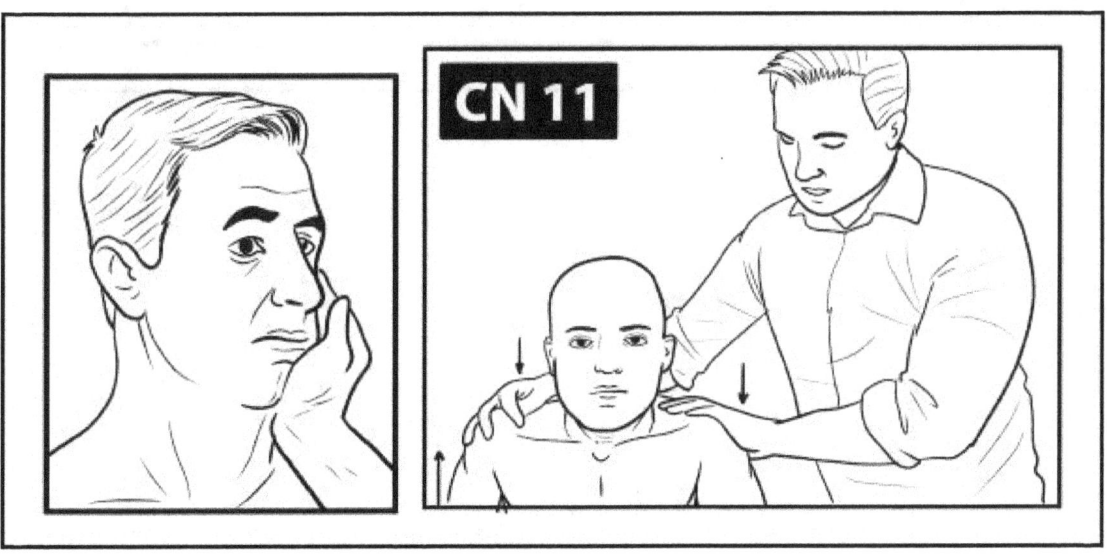

**Cranial Nerve Examination**

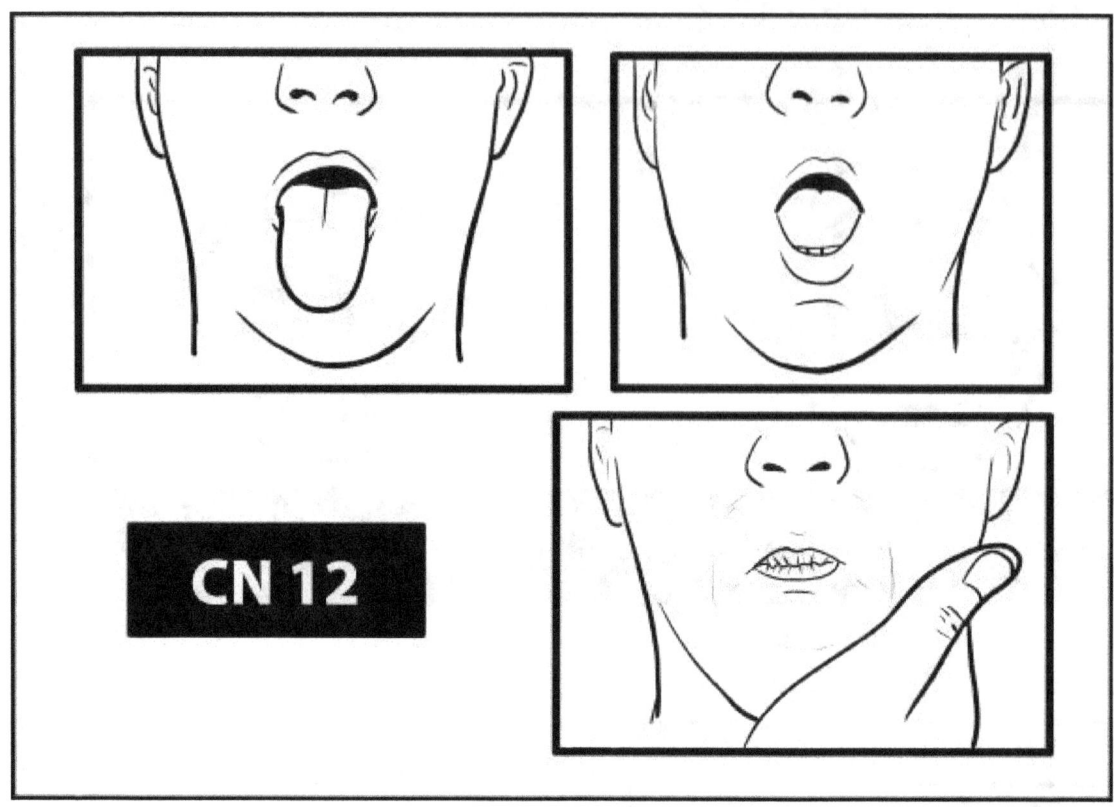

## Parkinson Examination

| | |
|---|---|
| **General** | 1. Pt at 45 degree bed, sleeves up, devices, walking aid<br>2. Hypomania = masked facies (akinesia)<br>3. Monotonous speech (Hypophonia)<br>4. Drooling (Akinesia)<br>5. Offer to examine CN 1: loss of sense of smell (early sign) |
| **Tremor** | • At rest<br>• 4 and 6 hertz (cycles per second)<br>• asymmetry<br>• Pill-rolling<br>• Worsen by stress (ask Pt to count backwards from 10 to 1)<br>• Diminished with postural (ask to stretch his arms out and spread fingers)<br>• Diminished with movement (do finger nose test) |
| **Rigidity** | • Check tone<br>• **Rigidity:**<br>- **Hypertonia & Without tremor:** lead pipe = continue resistance<br>- **Hypertonia With tremor:** cogwheel = intermittent change in tone with passive movement<br><br>| Rigidity | Spasticity |<br>|---|---|<br>| • Extrapyramidal lesions<br>• Uniform hypertonia (resistance) throughout the movement<br>• Velocity independent<br>• Example lead pipe | • Pyramidal tract (UMN lesion)<br>• Initial resistance with sudden release<br>• (Clasp knife)<br>• Velocity dependent (increase with speed)<br>• jjes+++ weakness, hyperreflexia |<br><br>- exacerbated by asking Pt move the contralateral limb (tap his contralateral knee with his contralateral hand) |

## Parkinson Examination

| | |
|---|---|
| **Akinesia /bradykinesia (slow movement)** | - Finger tapping (play a piano)<br>- Opening and closing the fist<br>- Pinching movement<br>- Pronating and supinating the wrist<br>- Tapping with heels |
| **Postural Disturbances (Gait)** *high risk of fall stand by the patient | - shuffling Gait:<br>- Difficulty in standing up and initiated the first movement<br>- Movement speed increases after starting the first few movement (festination)<br>- Loss of arm swing<br>- Short steps<br>- Flexed posture (Simian posture)<br>- (Propulsion) or backward (Retropulsion). |
| **Special Tests** | 1. **Retropulsion or forced pull back test**<br>  a. Stand behind the Pt<br>  b. Pt eyes must be opened<br>  c. Ask Pt to maintain his/her stability while you pull the Pt from the shoulder toward you<br>- **POSITIVE**:<br>  - Retropulsion<br>  - Take few steps backwards<br>- **Micrographic**: (bradykinesia)<br>  - Ask Pt to write a sentence<br><br>2. **Glabellar reflex**<br>  a. Tap on Pt's forehead.<br>  b. In normal Pt blinking will disappear after few tapping<br>  c. Parkinson will persist |
| **The End** | - **Rule out differentials:**<br>  - Lewy body dementia: by doing MMSE<br>  - SPS: vertical gaze palsy (eye movement test)<br>  - Multiple system atrophy (hypotension, cerebellar examination)<br>  - Look at drugs charts (atypical antipsychotic)<br>  - offer to do full neurological examination & MSE (depression) |

❖ **Parkinsonian: (extrapyramidal diseases)**

# Parkinson Examination

- **TRAP**
  - Tremor, Rigidity, Akinesia, and Postural disturbances
  - Death of substantia nigra cells (midbrain) causes loss of dopamine
  - Biopsy: lewy body (hyaline inclusion bodies)
  - Early sign: loss of sense of smell (olfactory nerve), REM sleep behavior disorder (act out his dream), constipation

- **DD:**
  - **Lewy body dementia:**
  - Dementia
  - Visual hallucinations
  - Fluctuations in cognition

3. **Progressive Supranuclear palsy:**
   - **Vertical gaze palsy:** start with a downgaze palsy followed by up gaze palsy.    *will not look at the floor
   - **Axial rigidity:** neck and back as a result Pt will arched backward

   - **Multiple system atrophy (Shy-Drager syndrome)**
   - Autonomic dysfunction (BP instability + ED) + cerebellar signs + bowel/bladder dysfunction
   - **Corticobasal degeneration:**
   - AAA
   - Aphasia + alien limb phenomenon + apraxia

- **Treatment :**
  - Anticholinergic (Benztropine)
  - Amantadine
  - **Levodopa/carbidopa : most effective:** phenomenon)
    *SE:(Dyskinesia's ,on–off"
  - Dopamine agonist (Ropinirole, bromocriptine, Pramipexole)
  - Monoamine oxidase B
  - Inhibitors (Selegiline)
  - COMT(entacapone)
  - Deep brain stimulation of the subthalamic nucleus or globus pallidus

- **Rule out**
  - Pyramidal tract diseases by excluding: hyperreflexia clonus, extensor plantar upward movement
  - Peripheral nerve diseases: Areflexia, sensory loss, weakness

**Parkinson Examination**

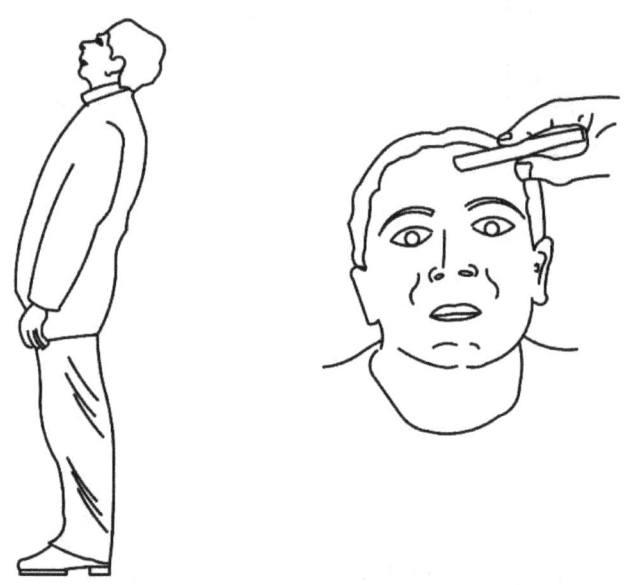

**Progressive Supranuclear palsy**

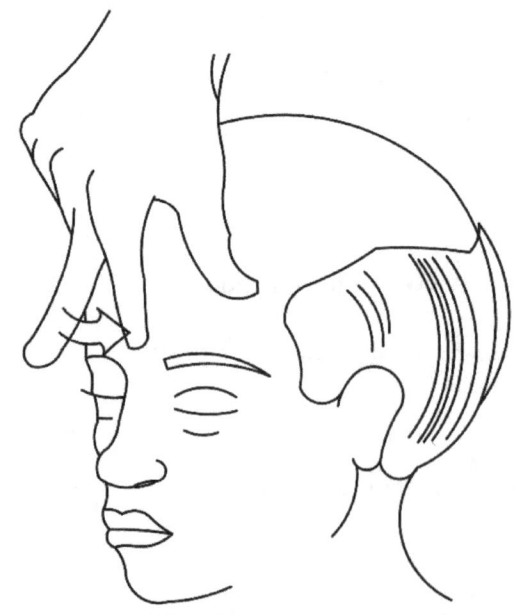

**Glabellar reflex**

## Parkinson Examination

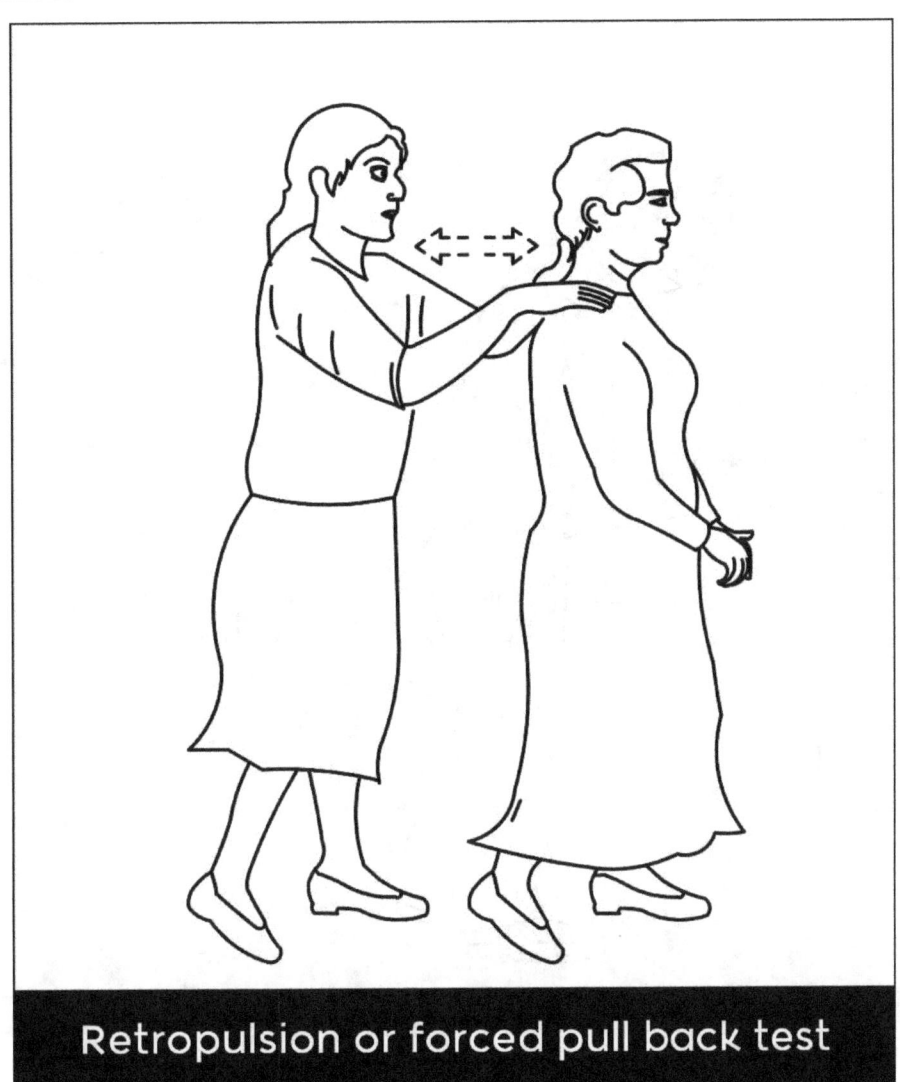

Retropulsion or forced pull back test

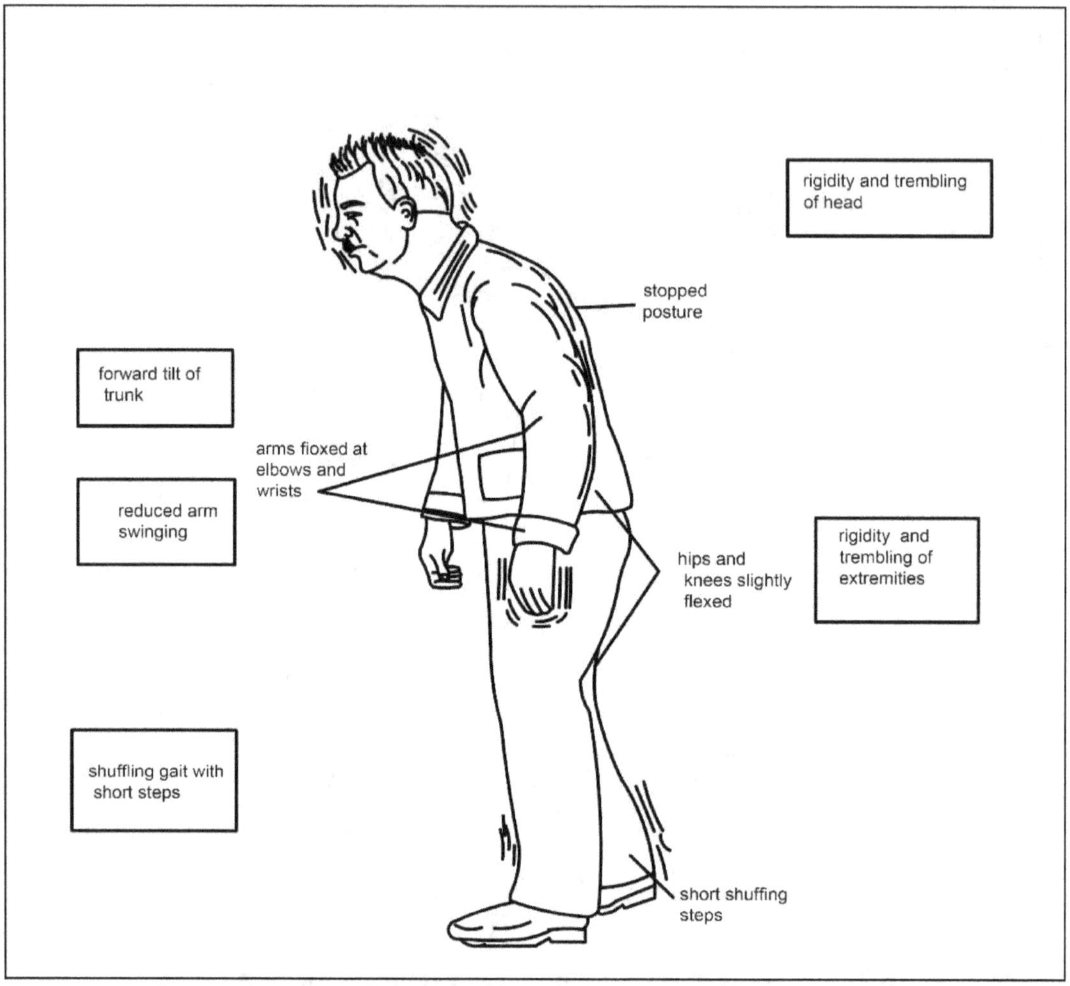

## Parkinson Examination

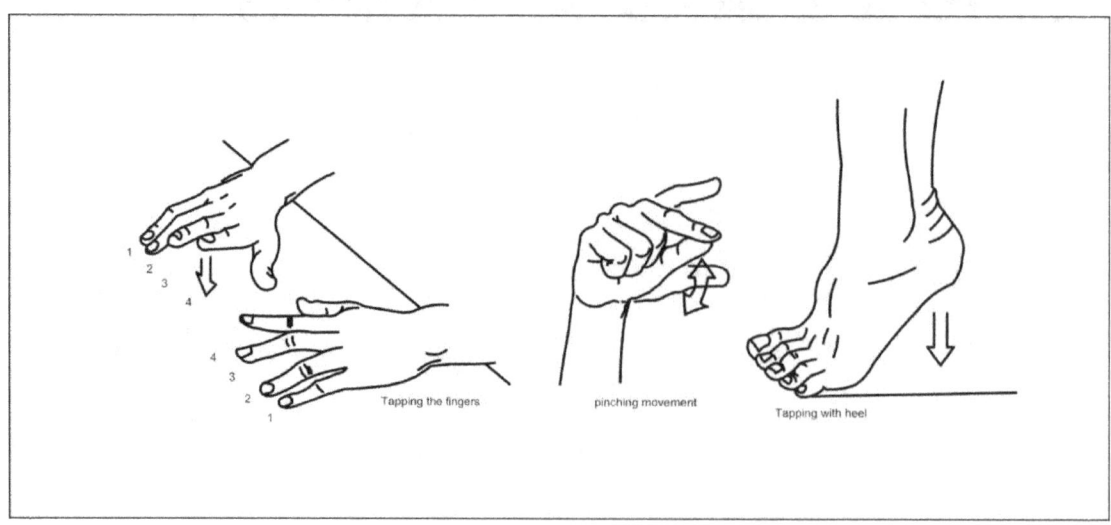

# Parkinson Examination

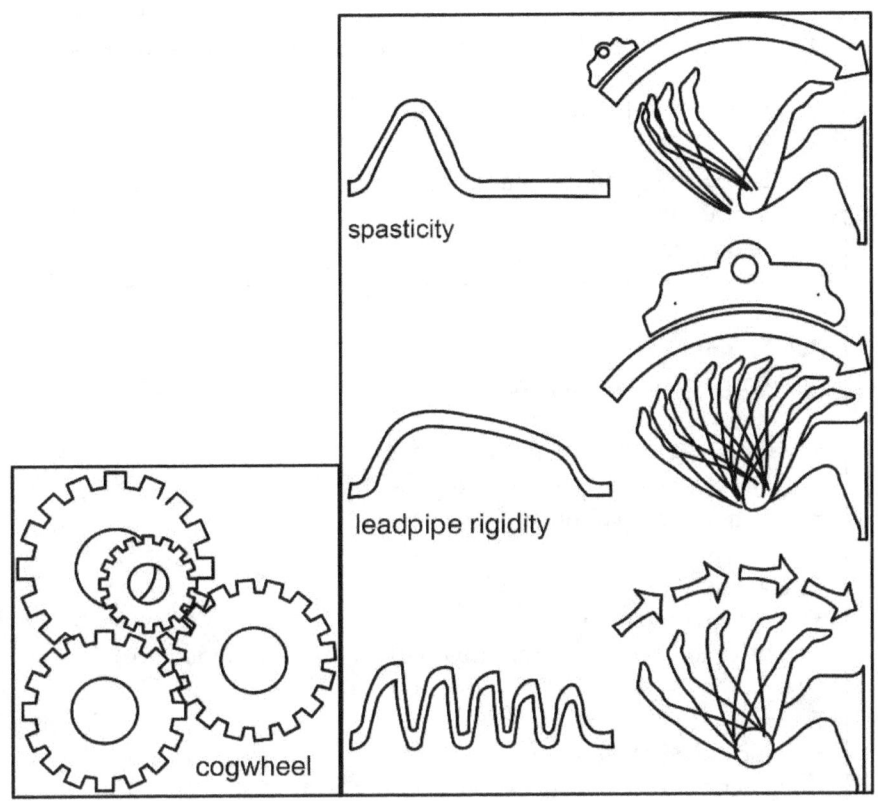

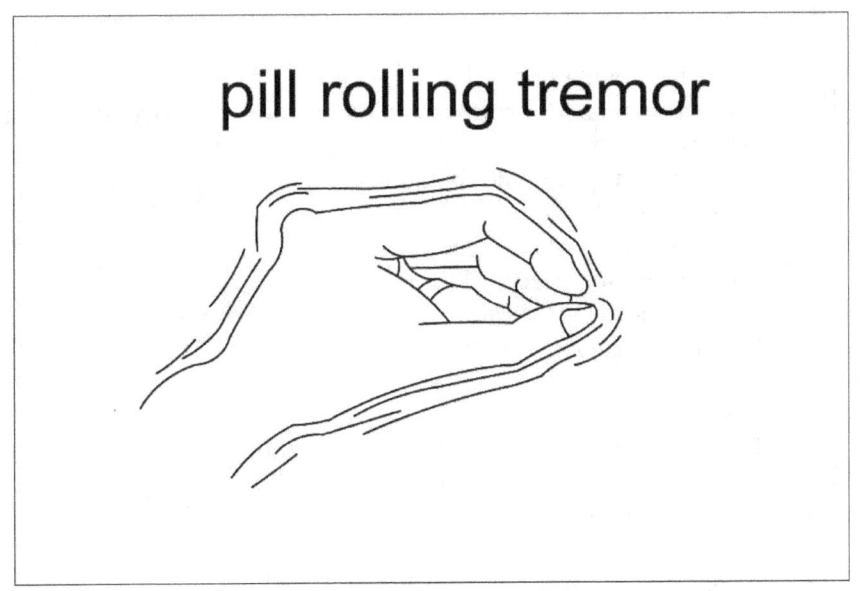

## Acromegaly Examination

| | |
|---|---|
| **General** | 1. Wash your hands, introduce yourself, gain consent, Rule out any Pain<br>2. Position at 45° supported with one pillow/chairs<br>3. Top is off<br>4. Devices & walking aid (arthritis), ECG(cardiomyopathy)<br>5. Voice (deep)<br>6. Shoe size |
| **Starting from Hands** | 1. **Hands:**<br>- Large hands & fingers<br>- Palm (sweaty &warm)<br>- Dorsal (coarse, thicken)<br>- Diabetic finger prick marks<br>- Signs of carpal tunnel syndrome<br><br>2. **Arms**<br>- BP (hypertension)<br>- offer to check proximal myopathy (shoulder abduction)<br><br>3. **Neck:**<br>- Increased JVP<br>- Goitre<br>- Skin tags (molluscum fibrosum): associated with colonic polyps<br>- Acanthosis Nigricans<br><br>4. **Face**<br>- Coarsened facial features<br>- Look from side for prominent supraorbital ridges (frontal bossing)<br>- large nose and lips<br>- Prognathism (prominent mandible/jaw)<br>- Widen of teeth<br>- Macroglossia (large tongue)<br>- Pituitary tumor effect:<br>- Visual fields (looking for bitemporal hemianopia)<br>- Papilloedema (increase ICP)<br><br>5. **Chest**<br>- Body hair and gynecomastia (high prolactin level may be secreted from the same pituitary tumor that secretin GH)<br>- Cardiomyopathy (cardiomegaly)<br>- Palpate apex beat: displaced apex<br>- Listen for murmur: dilated heart cause valve incomplete (AR, MR)<br>- Listen to lung bases (bibasal crepitations)<br><br>6. **Abdomen** |

**Acromegaly Examination**

|  |  |
|---|---|
|  | - Percuss or palpate Organomegaly (hepatomegaly or splenomegaly, nephromegaly)<br>- Testicular atrophy (high prolactin level)<br>- Legs<br>- Proximal myopathy (ask patient to stand with arms crossed)<br>- Peripheral oedema (CHF from cardiomyopathy)<br>- Osteartins (knee) |
| The End | • **Mention if the disease is active by these signs and symptoms:**<br>1. skin tags number<br>2. Sweating (sweat gland hypertrophy)<br>3. Glycosuria;<br>4. Visual field loss<br>5. Enlarging goitre;<br>6. Hypertension<br>• Capillary blood glucose<br>• Urine dip (glucose)<br>• ECG<br>• Sleep study (1 Sleep apnoea)<br>• Screening colonoscopy |

## ❖ Increased growth hormone:

a. Gigantism: pre puberty and fusion of growth plate
b. Acromegaly :post puberty and after the fusion of growth plates

- **Acromegaly:**
- **Due:**
a. Pituitary tumor releasing GH (mostly mixed with other hormone like prolactin)
b. Ectopic GHRH from pancreatic cancer or carcinoid

- **Diagnostic:**
- IGF-1
- Glucose tolerance test (GH will be high even after glucose)
- MRI(brain)

- **Treatment:**
- Transsphenoidal resection
- Dopamine agonists (Cabergoline)
- Somatostatin analogues (octreotide)
- GH antagonist (Pegvisomant)
- Radiation therapy (last resort)

## Acromegaly Examination

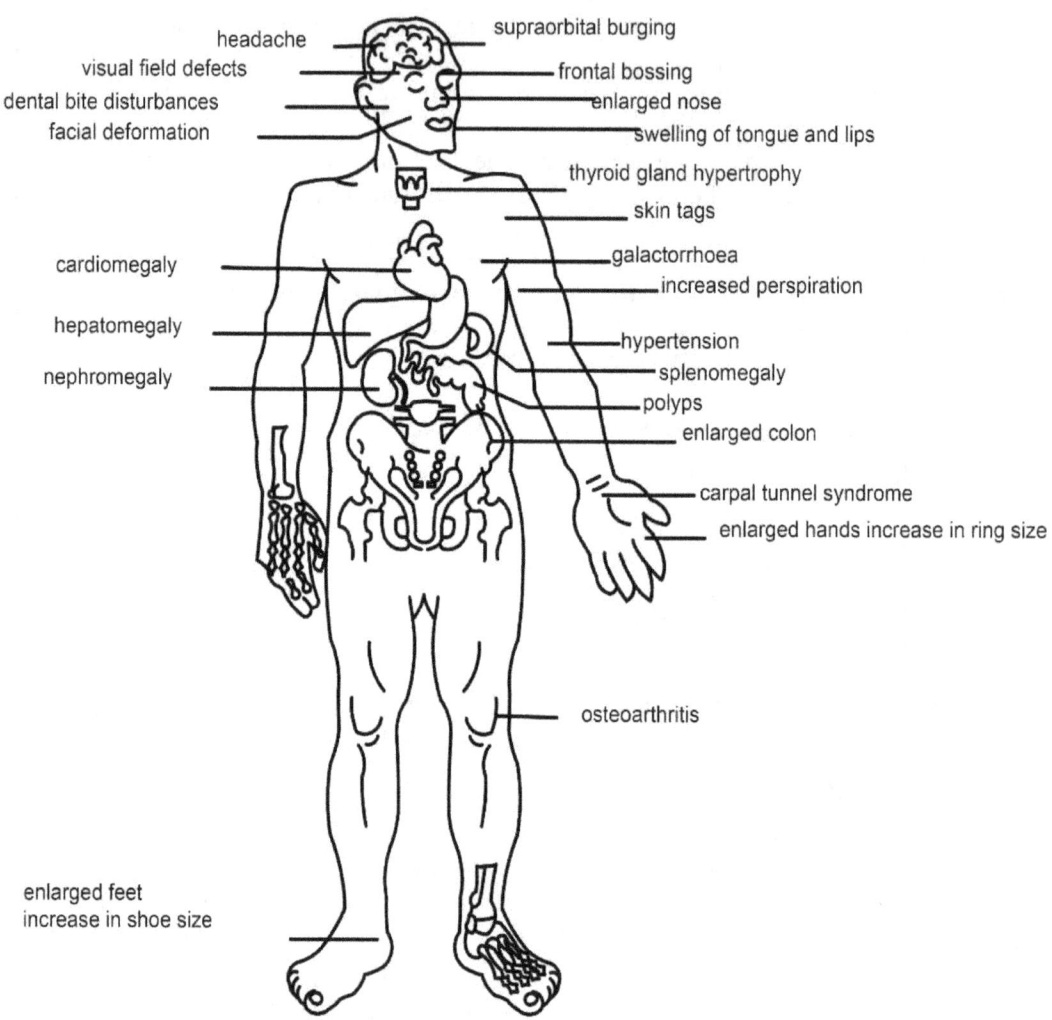

# Cushing Examination

| | |
|---|---|
| **General** | 1. Wash your hands, introduce yourself, Pt seated with top off or laying on a bed<br>2. Devices, medication (steroid)<br>3. From the end of the bed: central obesity, thinning of extremities, Striae (red), alert (steroid induced psychosis) |
| **Inspection** | 1. **Hand & arms:**<br>- Petechiae or ecchymosis (Easy bruising)<br>- Thin skinfold (Skin atrophy): can be measured= thickness less than 18 mm<br>- Proximal myopathy (weak shoulder abduction)<br>- Pigmentation (ACTH dependent Cushing syndrome)<br>- BP(hypertension)<br>2. **Face:**<br>- Acne Greasy skin<br>- Plethora<br>- Rounded face with visible vessel (thin skin)<br>- Hirsutism<br>- Visual field: (bitemporal hemianopia due ACTH releasing pituitary adenoma), papilledema<br>3. **Shoulder:**<br>- Supraclavicular fat pads (Buffalo hump)<br>4. **Abdomen:**<br>- Gynecomastia (adrenal pathology)<br>- Central obesity<br>- Striae(red)<br>5. **Spinal tenderness on palpation:**<br>- Osteoarthritis<br>6. **Hip examination for avascular necrosis**<br>- Legs: proximal myopathy |
| **The End** | - **Do bedside Tests:**<br>- Urine dipstick (glucose)<br>- Fasting blood glucose<br>- Dexa (osteoporosis) |

❖ **Cushing syndrome:**

## Cushing Examination

- **Causes:**
1. **ACTH dependent:**
a. Cushing disease (a pituitary adenoma
b. Ectopic ACTH production (small cell lung cancer

2. **Non-ACTH:**
a. Adrenal adenomas or carcinomas
b. Exogenous steroids(most common)

- **Investigations:**
- 24-hour measurement of free cortisol levels in urine
- Salivary cortisol level
- Low dose dexamethasone suppression test: if cortisol levels is still high after given dexamethasone =positive Cushing syndrome

 * ACTH is high in Cushing disease and ectopic source
 * ACTH is low in an adrenal adenoma (cortisol released from adrenal gland inhibit ACTH released from pituitary gland (negative feedback)

- **High dose dexamethasone suppression test:**
a. **If pituitary adenoma:** ACTH, cortisol levels will be suppressed do brain MRI
b. **If ectopic release the:** ACTH, cortisol level will still be high do chest x-ray &CT

- **Treatment:**
1. Transsphenoidal resection: Cushing diseases
2. Adrenal adenoma or carcinoma: adrenalectomy

# Renal Examination

| | |
|---|---|
| **General** | 1. Wash your hands and introduce yourself<br>2. Gain consent and rule out any pain<br>3. Pt positioned at 45-degree bed<br>4. Devices, peritoneal dialysis bags, central line, urinary (Foley) catheter<br>5. Uremia complications: alert and oriented(encephalopathy), excoriations(pruritus), colour(yellow), tachypnea (Respiratory compensation for metabolic acidosis)<br>6. Fluid over volume:(SOB, orthopnea) |
| **Hands & Arms** | • **Nails :**<br>a. Leukonychia (hypoalbumin)<br>b. Brown nail banding(CKD)<br>c. Beau's lines : grooved lines on fingernail(hypoalbuminemia)<br>d. Muehrcke's nails: transverse white line(hypoalbuminemia in nephrotic syndrome)<br>e. skin turgor (dehydration status , the slowest the skin unfolded the more dehydrated the patient )<br>f. capillary refill(normal if less than 2-3 sec)<br>g. prick needles marks(diabetes)<br>h. koilonychia(anemia)<br><br>• **Dorsal hand**: xanthomata(nephrotic syndrome and CKD causes hyperlipidemia)<br>• **Palm :**<br>a. Pallor of palmar creases<br>b. Flap (uremic encephalopathy)<br>c. If Pt has renal transplant (not on dialysis) check tremor (cyclosporine)<br>d. Offer to check pulses (tachycardia with dehydration)<br>e. BP (high in renal artery stenosis , ADPKD ,rejection ,CKD,nephritic syndrome)<br>f. Bruising in arms(platelet dysfunction due uremia)<br>g. skin lesion in arms: BCC, SCC(immunosuppressive drugs )<br>h. Parathyroid Preimplantation in Forearm |
| | • **Inspection :**<br>• **Site** : radiocephalic below cubital fossa(above writs) , above cubital fossa (brachiocephalic )<br>• **Shape** : (cylindrical/longitudinal with or without localized dilation indicate pseudoaneurysm)<br>• **Size( cms)**<br>• **Pulsatile** |

# Renal Examination

| | |
|---|---|
| **AV Fistula Examination** | - **Needelig mark (being used) or dressing**<br>- **Erythema(infection)**<br>- **Scar (size and transverse or vertical)**<br>- Feel for tenderness(infection)<br>- Temperature with back of your hand (infection)<br>- Start palpating from the distal part to proximal part (near neck )<br>    -Comment if its palpable through veins or not<br>    -Find the thrill(vibration/buzzing feeling)=AV anastomosis)<br>- Auscultate for bruit (mechanical sound)=patent<br>- Impalpable thrill and without bruit auscultation (non-functioning AV fistula)<br><br>- **Special Test :**<br>- **augmentation test (check outflow):**<br>- Rule out shoulder pain<br>- Ask Pt to raise arm<br>- If the lump becomes less prominence (outflow is not obstructed)<br>- **Inflow Test :**<br>- Find the thrill (vibration )<br>- With one hand move 1 or 2 cms proximally and press here with other hand feel with other hand feel over the anatomies (thrill is replaced with pulsation )<br>- **Allen Test:**<br>- To rule out steal syndrome , this examination usually done pre AV fistula made to if radial or ulnar nerve in compensate (that indicate the AVF is not suitable to be done in this arm) |
| **Head and Neck** | - **Eye:**<br>- Lemon tinge<br>- Pallor conjunctiva mouth<br>- Uraemic fetor(smell breath)<br>- Gingival hyperplasia (calcineurin inhibitors)<br>- **Neck**<br>- Parathyroidectomy scar(tertiary hyperparathyroidism treatment )<br>- JVP(volume overload from oliguria, hypoalbuminemia )<br>- Auscultate for carotid artery bruits (atherosclerosis diseases may hint to renal artery atherosclerosis)*<br>- Offer to auscultate heart (MVP causes AR )+++ADPKD<br>- Pericardial rub (pericarditis from uremia)<br>- Central hemodialysis catheter or scar:<br>1. Usually internal jugular vein (from angle of mandible to middle part of clavivale )<br>2. Complication :arrhythmia , pneumothorax , hematoma |

# Renal Examination

| | |
|---|---|
| **Abdomen: patient must lie flat and supported by one pillow and arms by side** <br><br> *same exposure as abdominal examination | ▪ **Inspection** : Ideally lie flat <br> a. **Scar** :nephrectomy open or laparoscopic (flank),Rutherford Morrison (iliac area above inguinal ligament) <br> b. **Tenckhoff catheter dialysis or scars**(near umbilicus) <br> c. **abdominal distension** (ascites) <br> * If you see scar ask Pt to cough for incisional hernia <br><br> • **Palpate the 9 areas of abdomen** (rule out mass , tenderness (peronitisis),obstruction ) <br><br> ▪ **Kidney Ballot :** <br> • Put your left hand under patient's back and press forward (specifically under the loin area not under ribs )and your right hand must be over anterior abdomen lateral to rectus muscle <br> • Ask the Pt to take deep breath in <br> • At peak of inspiration press firmly with your right hand <br> • If you feel the kidney then ask Pt to breath out feel the kidney slide back to its place push it between your left and right hand <br> • **Palpate transplanted kidney** <br> - (describe as LUMP ) see below to differentiate between it and spleen <br> * immunosuppression side effects (hirsutism, cushingoid appearance ,skin cancer) <br> • liver palpation for hepatomegaly (ADPKD) <br> • Shifting dullness/fluid thrill <br> • Auscultate renal bruit (systolic and diastolic murmur) |
| **Legs** | • Oedema |
| **The End** | • **Offer to examine :** <br> • **Costovertebral angle :** <br> a. Dullness = mass <br> b. Tenderness = pyelonephritis <br><br> ▪ **Do fully examination to diabetic Pt :** <br> • Fundoscopy :diabetic retinopathy, hypertensive retinopathy <br> • Diabetic foot <br> • To examine testicls for varicocele—tumor thrombus in the renal vein or left RCC <br> • Lung and spine for RCC metastasis to bone and lung <br> • DRE: prostate pathology cause hydronephrosis <br> • Urinalysis |

## Renal Examination

| Spleen | Kidney |
|---|---|
| <ul><li>Spleen notch</li><li>Can cross midline</li><li>Can't get above</li><li>Move down on inspiration</li><li>Not ballotable</li><li>Splenic rub</li><li>Dullness</li></ul> | <ul><li>No notch</li><li>Never cross midline</li><li>May get above</li><li>Doesn't move with respiration</li><li>Ballotable</li><li>No rub</li><li>Resonance (underlie colon)</li></ul> |

❖ **Autosomal Dominant (ADPKD):**
- SXS: Loin Pain hematuria, HTN
- Complication: cerebral aneurysm(berry)&SAH ,liver cyst , MVP, diverticulosis

❖ **Renal Cell Carcinoma Triad:**
- Flank pain, hematuria, and flank mass

❖ **Kidney mass:**

1. **Unilateral**
- RCC
- Solitary cyst
- Adrenal tumors
- Hydronephrosis
- Abscess (Perinephric).
- ADPKD with asymmetric enlargement
- Renal vein thrombosis
- Hypertrophy (following contralateral nephrectomy)

2. **Bilateral**
- ADPKD
- bilateral hydronephrosis or pyonephrosis
- bilateral RCC
- renal vein thrombosis (bilateral)
- Systemic (amyloid, acromegaly)

❖ **AKI :**
- Stratified by RIFLE system
- SXS:
- Fluid over volume (increased JVP ,dyspnea ,bibasal crepitations ,oedema)
- Hyperkaliemia:(muscle weakness , arrhythmia)
- Oliguria
- Metabolic acidosis
1. **Post renal (large bladder ):** stone , BPH, neurogenic atony diagnosed by USS and treat with Foley catheter
2. **Pre renal :** decreased renal perfusion :

## Renal Examination

a. Decreased cardiac output(MI , CHF , cardiac tamponade)
b. Volume depletion :(bleeding ,burn ,GIT loss by vomiting and diarrhea)
c. peripheral vasodilation(anaphylaxis, sepsis ,hepatorenal syndrome)
d. Drugs (NSAID, aspirin)**
e. Renal artery stenosis

- **Physiology** :Decreased in renal perfusion will cause decreased GFR , however compensated system start to increase GFR by:
1. Prostaglandin cause afferent vasodilation
2. Angiotensin II causes efferent vasoconstriction

- These two steps assure that GFR is mainsted and both drugs affect them
- NSAID inhibit Prostaglandin
- ACEI inhibit Angiotensin II

1. **Intrarenal :**
a. ATN(muddy brown cast)
b. nephrotoxic drugs (contrast gentamicin ,rhabdomyolysis )
c. Acute Interstitial Nephritis: medication allergy , infection
d. Tubular Blockage: by virus drugs( acyclovir ,indinavir ) ,stones (UA ,calcium)

|  | **Prerenal Failure** | **Intrarenal** |
|---|---|---|
| **Fractional Na+ excretion** | low | high |
| **BUN/Cr** | high | low |
| **Urinary Sodium** | low | high |
| **Urine Osmolality** | high | low |

❖ **Dialysis types:**
- **Indications** for dialysis or renal transplant :
a. Hyperkalemia(refractory)
b. Metabolic acidosis(refractory)
c. Fluid over volume (refractory)
d. Uremic symptoms,(N/V ,pericarditis ,neuropathy , encephalopathy)
e. GFR (below 15 or 10)
- **Complication:**
a. N/v
b. Muscle cramp
c. Hypotension
d. Amyloidosis
e. Dialysis disequilibrium syndrome(cerebral edema)
f. First-use syndrome
- **Hemodialysis:**

# Renal Examination

- 3 time per week for 4 hrs.
- Treatment adequacy is shown by urea clearance
- Refer to check for vascular access if serum Cr is >4 mg/dl or the GFR is <25 mL/min.

- **Methods:**
1. **Arteriovenous (AV) fistula** (longer life time, less complications)
- **Types:**
a. Radial A+ cephalic V=radiocephalic (Brescia-Cimino)
b. Brachial A to cephalic V = brachiocephalic

- NO Venipuncture or BP to be done at AV fistula hand

- **Advantages of hemodialysis.**
- More efficient than peritoneal dialysis.
- High flow rates and efficient dialyzers
- shorten the period of time required for dialysis.

- **Complications :**
- Hypotension ( rapid fluid removal )
- Hypo-osmolality

- **AV Fistula:**
- Stenosis
- Thrombosis
- limb ischemia (steal syndrome)
- Air embolism
- high output failure : blood flow>1000 ml/min

- **Fistula Maturation**
- **Rule of 6's**
- 6 weeks old
- 6 mm deep
- 6 mm fistula diameter
- 600ml per min flow

2. **AV graft**
- If vascular access is not suitable do graph
  i. **Pros**: ready to be used in few 3 weeks
  ii. **Cons**: higher rate of thrombosis, life time is 2 years

- **Types:**
- Synthetic tube connect artery to vein
- Straight graft connect radial A and the basilica V
- Loop graft connect brachial A and the basilica V


3. **Catheter (Central)**

## Renal Examination

- Central venous access to internal jugular
- Tunneled (longer use), non-tunneled(acute injury not more than use 2 weeks )
- Continuous venovenous hemofiltration by central venous
- Access for unstable Pt.

- **Complication:**
- **Infection:** Staphylococcus aureus
- Remove the catheter and reintroduce after blood culture is negative and afebrile for 2 days
- Bleeding
- Air embolism

4. **Peritoneal Dialysis :**
- **Limitation :**
a. Hernia (repair before do it)
b. Abdominal adhesion(history of multiple abdominal surgery)
c. Elderly , rheumatic hands(difficulty to perform it)

- **Types:**
- By Tenckhoff catheter;
- Continuous ambulatory peritoneal dialysis (capd) :4 times daily
- Automated peritoneal dialysis:(night time from itself)
- Hyperglycemia and hypertriglyceridemia.

- **Complication:**
- **Peritonitis:**
- Asymptomatic (cloudy dialysate)
- Abdominal pain ,fever
- Do Gram stain , cell count ,culture of the dialysate
- Peritonitis: WCC>100/µL&>50% PMN
- Do not remove catheter
- Treat with AB
- Constipation: laxative
- Catheter migration

### ❖ Kidney Transplant

- **Contradictions:**
- Active occult infections
- Active Occult malignancies
- Cardiac/pulmonary failure
  **\*\*relative contradiction if Pt with history of psychiatry diseases or history of non-compliant with drugs

- **Screen recipient for :**
- HIV , EBV ,CMV ,hepatitis B and C

## Renal Examination

- **Screen for tumor according to age and sex:**
  - Female : Pap smear, mammogram
  - Male : PSA. ,FOBT

- **Immunosuppression**: Three regime:
  A. Induction(acutely post-transplant)
  B. Maintenance for life
  C. Anti-Rejection (acute attack of rejection)
- **examples:**
  - Tacrolimus (calcineurin inhibitor) :SE (DM,HTN ,nephrotoxic
  - Cyclosporine(calcineurin inhibitor):SE(gum hypertrophy ,HTN , hirsutism ,hyperkalemia)
  - Prednisone: Cushing syndrome (DM ,acne , poor wound healing ,Wt. gain ,cataract , myopathy ,osteoporosis)

- **Post-transplant side effects**
  - SCC in skin and cervical
  - Cystic kidney disease and renal cell carcinoma in native kidney
  - Renal artery stenosis
  - Post-transplant lymphoproliferative disorder (PTLD)
     -Infection

- **Transplant rejection:** Increase Cr/BUN ,oliguria , HTN
1. Hyperacute
   - HLA ,ABO mismatch
   - Causing thrombosis of graft vessel

2. Acute
   - Weeks to months*
   - Timing is not the answer , biopsy is the answer
   - T CELL immune mediated attack to the organ
   - Present as tenderness, increasing Creatine
   - Do biopsy (t-lymphocyte infiltration of vessels)
   - Give steroid , antilymphocyte

3. Chronic rejection :years
   - Interstitial fibrosis and tubular
   - Atrophy causing decreasing in function

- **Post-transplant check**
  - BP
  - RFT
  - Fasting Lipid and glucose
  - calcineurin inhibitor level
  - BK polyomavirus
  - PCR(CMV or EBV)
❖ **Nephritic Syndrome:**

## Renal Examination

- Proteinuria (≥3.5 g/d), edema, hypoalbuminemia, and hyperlipidemia ,frothy urine ,hypercoagulable state due to loss of antithrombin ,iron resistant microcytic hypochromic anemia , loss of Vitamin D

- **Primary cause**
a. Minimal Change Disease
b. Focal and Segmental Glomerulosclerosis (FSGS)
c. Membranous nephropathy
- **Secondary:**
a. DM (Kimmelstiel-Wilson lesions)
b. Amyloid
c. Lupus nephritis(cause both nephrotic and nephritic)

- **Nephritic Syndrome:**
- Hematuria, red cell casts, azotemia, variable proteinuria, oliguria, edema, and hypertension
- **Primary:**
a. Post-infectious Glomerulonephritis
b. IgA Nephropathy(HSP)

## ❖ CKD:

- GFR <60 mL/min +/- kidney damage for ≥3 months Causes:
- DM
- HTN
- ADPKD
- Glomerular disease
- GMN ,SLE ,amyloid
- Recurrent acute renal failure
- Vascular : renal artery stenosis ,vasculitis
- Interstitial nephritis

- **Severity is Graded by :**
a. eGFR
b. Albuminuria(the higher the worst )

- **Complications:**
- **Early :**anemia(normochromic normocytic) ,HTN
- **Late:** :hyperphosphatemia
- **MAD HUNGER:**
a. Metabolic Acidosis
b. Dyslipidemia (especially increased triglycerides)
- Hyperkalemia
- Uremia- clinical syndrome marked by increased BUN and creatinine
- Nausea and anorexia
- Pericarditis

## Renal Examination

- Asterixis
- Encephalopathy
- Platelet dysfunction(bleeding)
- Na+/water retention (CHF, pulmonary edema, hypertension)
- Growth retardation and developmental delay (in children)
- Erythropoietin failure (anemia)
- Renal osteodystrophy
- **Anemia:**

- **Bone disease in CKD:**

*Active form of Vitamin D is made in kidney by 1-alpha-hydroxylase

- low Vitamin D causes low calcium
- Phosphate is not removed by injured kidney
- High serum phosphate and low calcium causes high PTH

  - **Renal osteodystrophy**
    - Bone changes
    a. Osteomalacia
    b. Osteitis fibrosa cystica (secondary hyperparathyroidism): subperiosteal erosions, phalangeals ,skull (pepperpot skull)
    C. Osteosclerosis (rugger-jersey spine)

- **X-ray :**
- Osteopenia(early)
- Salt and pepper skull
- Subperiosteal resorption (radial aspects of middle phalanges )
- bone sclerosis
- (rugger-jersey spine)
- Atherosclerosis
- Cardiovascular disease is mostly the cause of death.

❖ **Hyperkalemia:**

- Weakness and paralysis

- **Causes:**
1. Renal failure
2. Extracellular shift (from inside cell into blood):
- Acidosis ,Beta blocker ,Rhabdomyolysis
3. Digoxin, Acei ,nsaid ,beta blocker

- **Tall peaked T waves**
- Loss of P waves
- Widening of QRS
- Sine wave, ventricular
- Arrhythmia, asystole

- **Managed by:**
- C BIG K (calcium gluconate, bicarbonate, insulin, glucose, kayexalate)

# Renal Examination

- **Renal artery stenosis :**
- Elderly is atherosclerosis
- Young female is **fibromuscular dysplasia**

## ❖ Indications for a Foley Catheter
- Retention
- Obstruction
- Urine output monitoring
- Diagnostic purposes
- Incontinence
- Imaging study
- Monitor Urine Output

- **Contradiction :**
- Urethral injury (blood at meatus , high riding prostate)

# Renal Examination

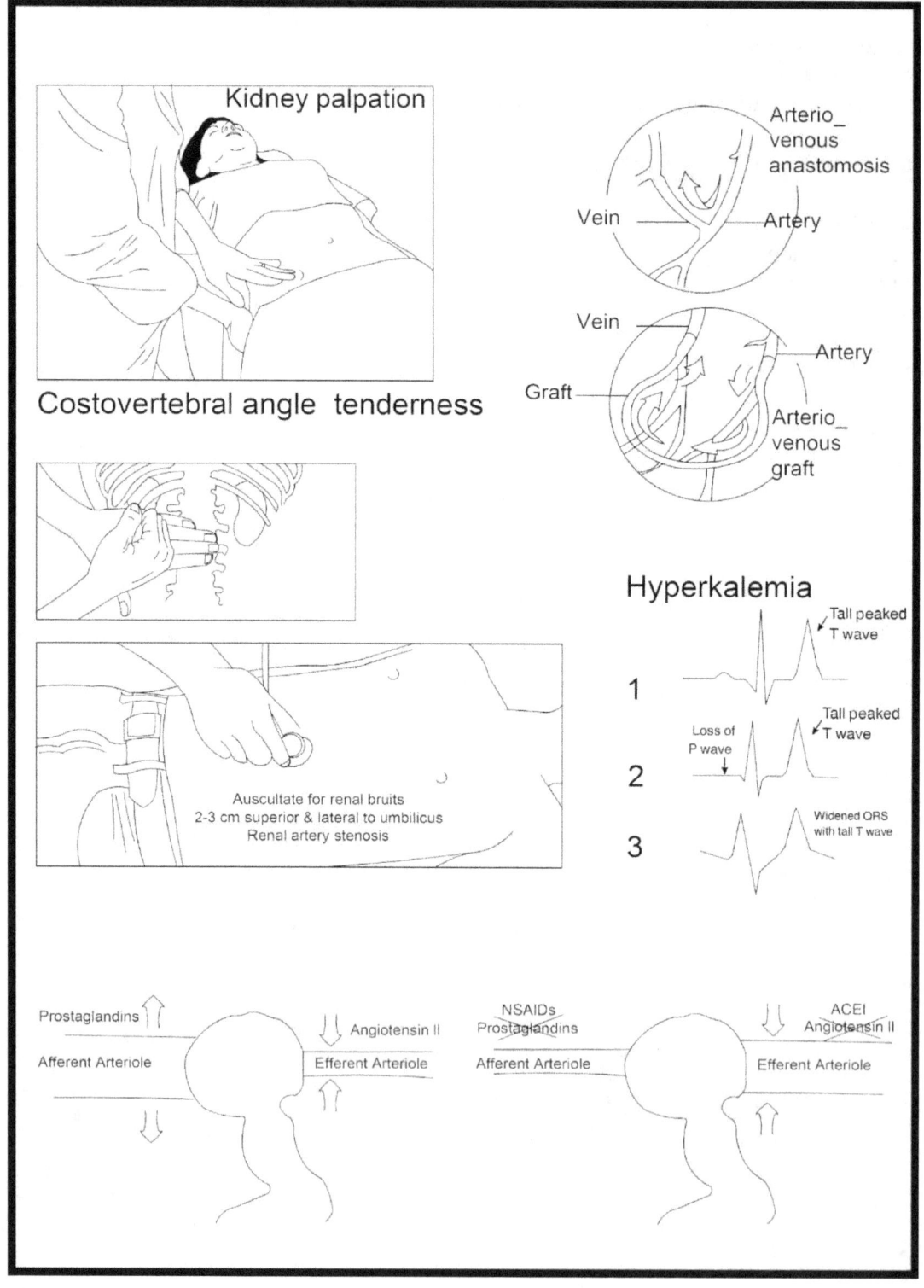

# Renal Examination

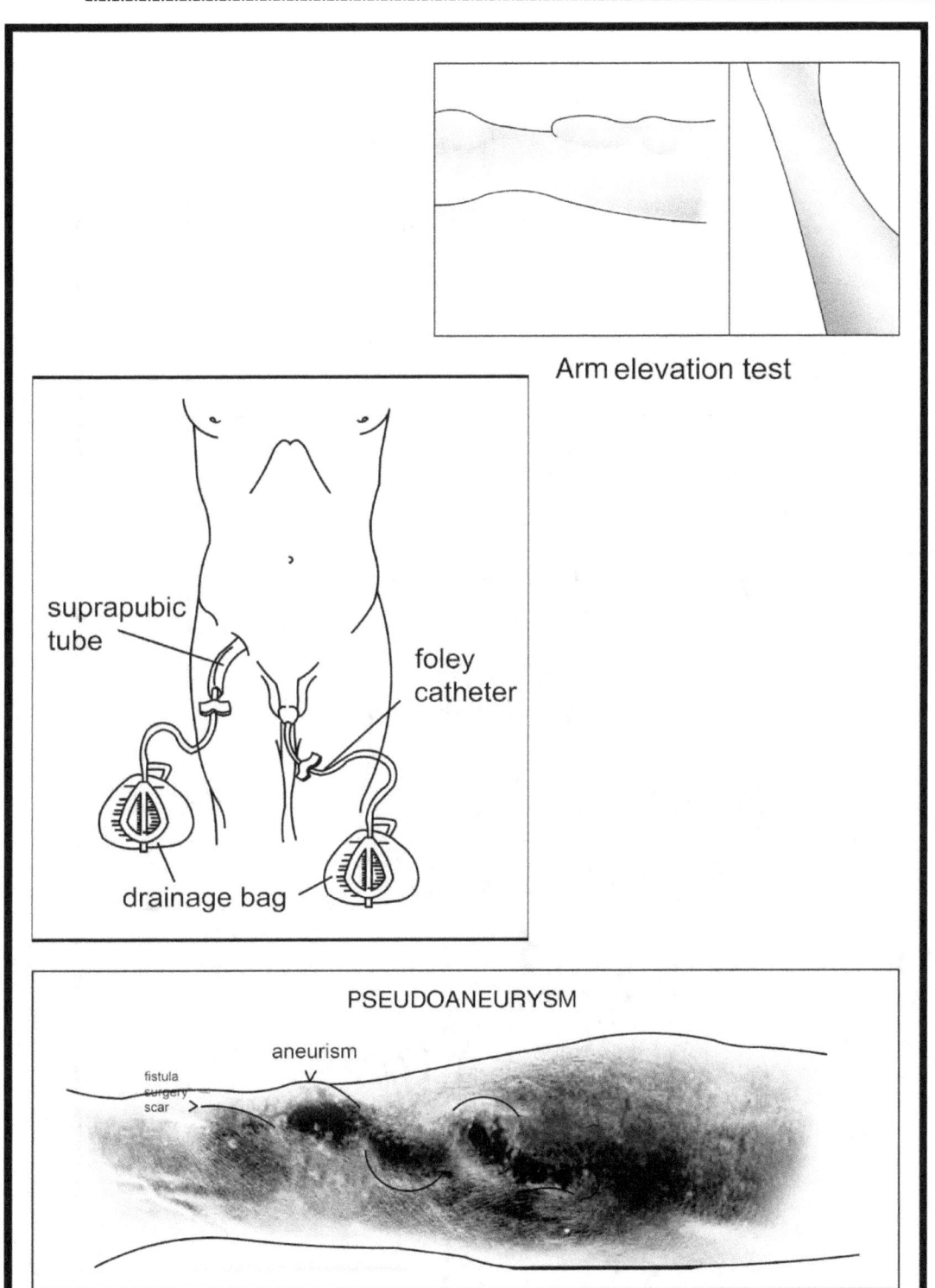

201

# Renal Examination

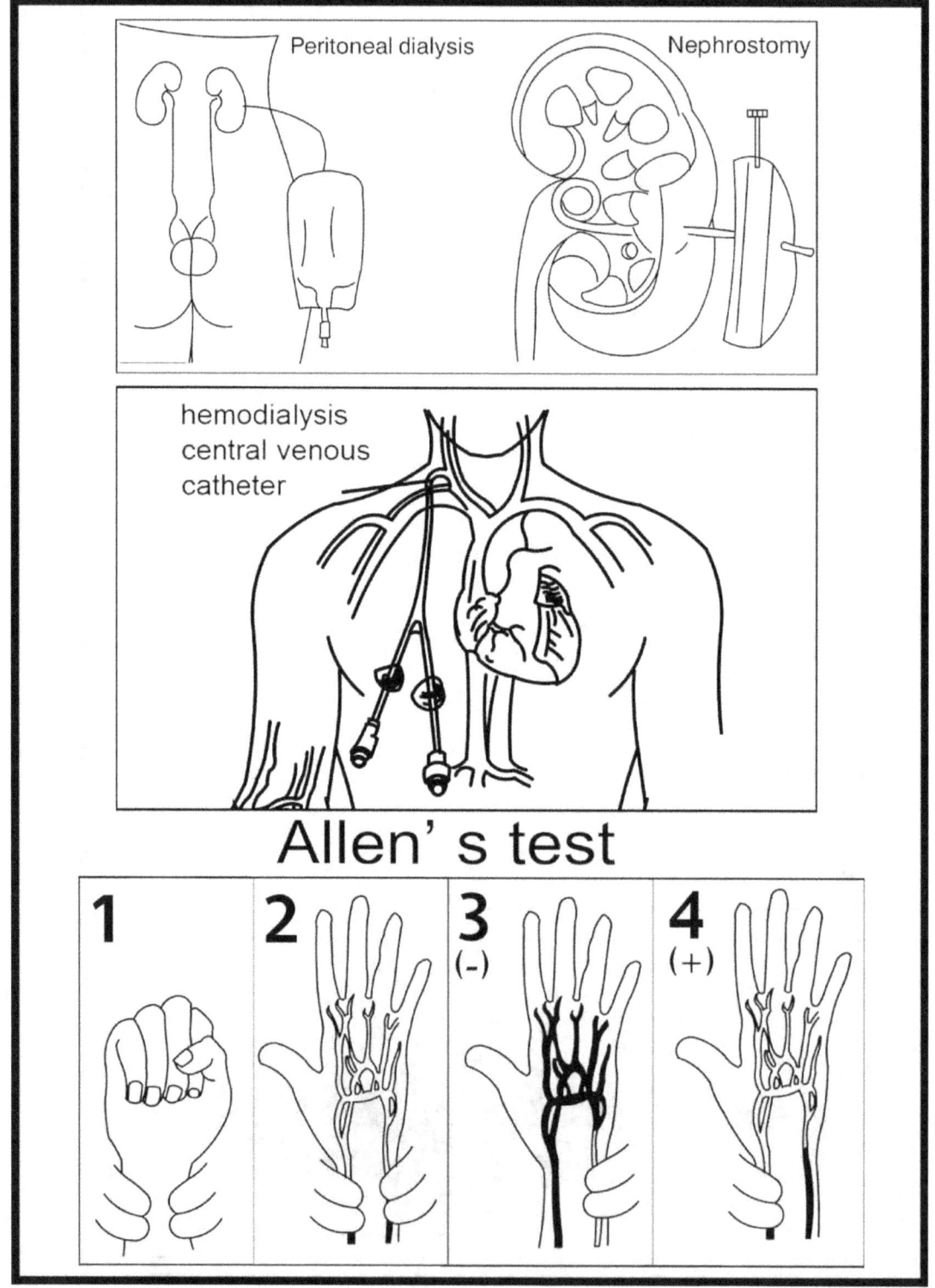

# Renal Examination

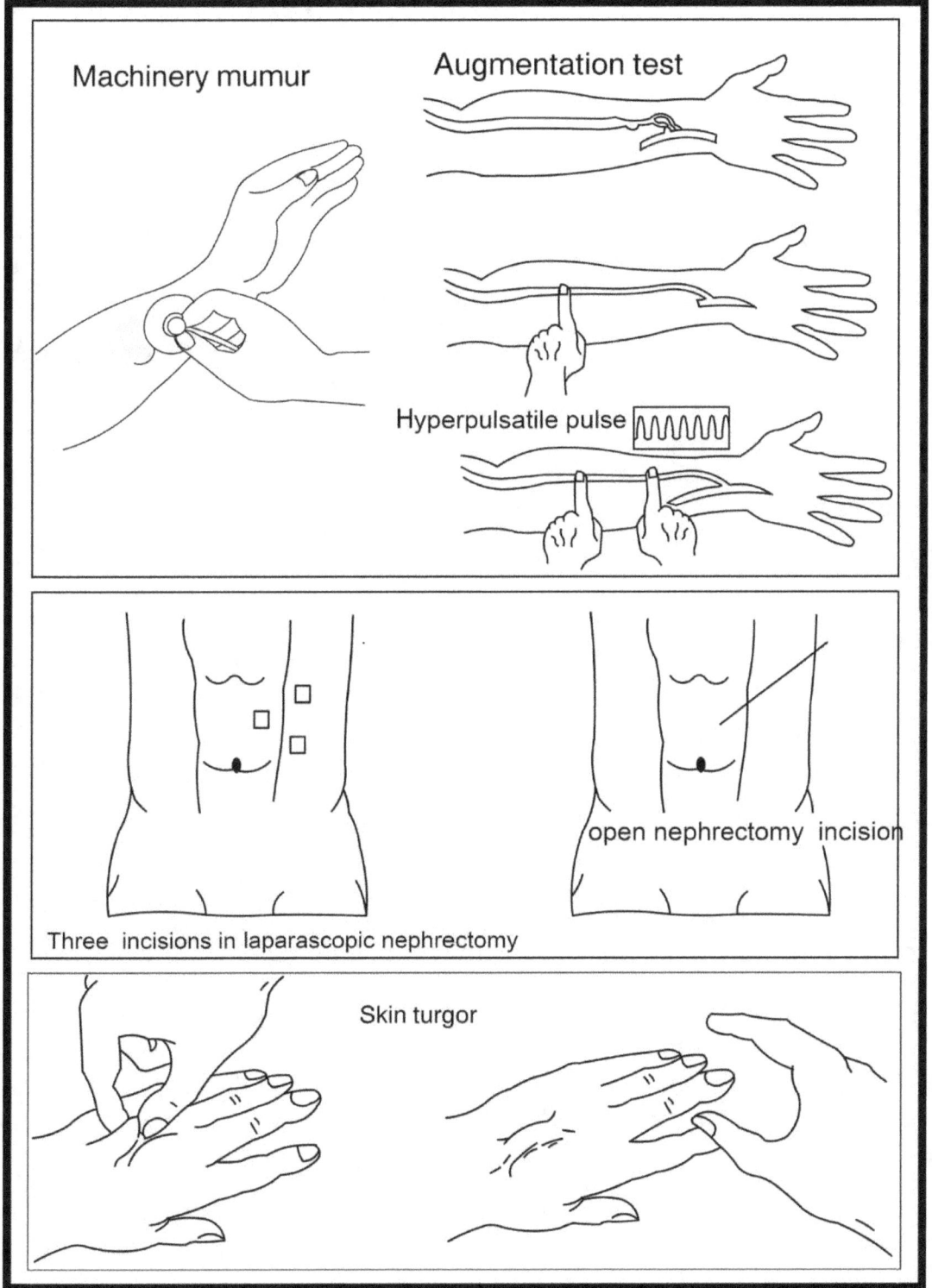

www.ingramcontent.com/pod-product-compliance
Lightning Source LLC
Chambersburg PA
CBHW080958170526
45158CB00010B/2834